From Archaea into Humans

A step-by-step guide

Dr. Erol A. Faruk

Copyright © 2020 Erol A. Faruk

All rights reserved

CONTENTS

Acknowledgements

About the Author

Introduction 4

1. **Earth's formation and initial life** 6

   Characterisation of life - first lifeforms - evidence for ancient bacteria - how bacteria live - DNA function and replication - DNA codons and amino acids - DNA **vs** RNA - origins of DNA and RNA - the RNA World - cyanobacteria and photosynthesis - oxygen rise in atmosphere.

2. **Complex life initiation** 16

   The Ediacarans - Cambrian Explosion - cellular presence of mitochondria - chemical energy production - large creatures possible - origin of mitochondria - prokaryotes vs eukaryotes - endosymbiosis - significance of the archaea - sea beds and alkaline vents - origin of plants - the Tree of Life.

3. **The evolutionary process** 24

   Dog varieties from wolf origin - simple eukaryotes - life's timeline - Paleozoic Era (ancient life) - Mesozoic Era (middle life) - Cenozoic Era (new life) - Earth's geological time scale - mass extinction events - rise of mammals - mammal characteristics - the Great Ape family - human evolution - ape/human differences - human brain development - the aging of life.

4. **The human genome and its quirks** 39

   23 Pairs of chromosomes - mitosis - trisomy disorders - gene coding errors - TP53 gene - body development genes - significance of sexual coupling - meiosis.

5. **Epilogue** 46

   Why only Earth? - Goldilocks zone of solar system - exoplanets - carbon-based life - Panspermia - intelligent alien life? - Summary - ubiquitous nature of chromosomes - Indian munkjac anomaly - DNA concordance among life.

Acknowledgements

I wish to thank all those websites that have provided the illustrations and informative links that appear in this book, and have ensured that each is properly referenced in order for readers to visit and appreciate for themselves.

I would also like to acknowledge the outstanding scientific research that has led to the elucidation of life's story so far that I have summarised here.

Finally I would like to thank the many authors whose detailed and extensive books on biological evolution have spurred me to write this concise version in order to facilitate the topic's comprehension by the general population.

About the Author

I was born in London, UK, from Turkish parents who emigrated from the island of Cyprus in 1948. After acquiring an early interest in amateur astronomy, I became eager to learn about science topics generally - in particular chemistry - and received my first degree followed by a PhD in that subject from Queen Mary College, London University. This was followed up with post-doctoral research positions at Oxford and Nottingham universities, before I took up full-time employment in 1979 as a pharmaceutical development chemist at Beecham Pharmaceuticals. This company subsequently merged and grew to become GlaxoSmithKline PLC in the year 2000. After retiring, my scientific interest focussed upon how life established itself as we now experience it, and found the story so compelling that I decided to write this book on the subject. I sincerely hope that the reader will also find the story as illuminating and interesting as I do.

Introduction

We live in a highly sophisticated 21st Century society in which a large proportion of the world's population are still only superficially aware of the scientific progress made in determining how life started on Earth and how humans eventually became the dominant intelligent species of (complex) animal life that exists today. I refer to 'complex' life because the story inevitably begins with the formation of simple bacterial life that we also co-habit with on this planet. The trigger for the conversion of this simple form into our complex one around two billion years ago is a remarkable story in itself, which needs to be known more widely.

This guide is not meant to be thorough in its review, but more of a concise description of the main elements, on which the reader is invited to seek further information as needed from the hyperlinks included.

The vital importance of something called 'evidence'

How do we know if something is true or not? Today, if an unusual event has happened and claimed to be true, people will want to see it for themselves. For example, if a volcano erupts in a remote island there will usually be film taken of the spectacle by camera men who will have ventured close by, and the film then circulated and watched by millions on their television screens. But what about events that have occurred a very long time ago? A characteristic of living things is that when they die they usually leave a solid residue (e.g. bones or fossils) that can be dug up much later and presented as evidence of their existence. In this way we know, for example, that huge creatures called dinosaurs once roamed the Earth millions of years ago.

But in the same way, we also know that a creature called the unicorn (i.e. a type of horse with a single horn on its forehead) is untrue, because the bones of such a creature have <u>never</u> been found. Its mythical origin is believed to have arisen from ancient Greek traveller descriptions of a similar creature likely to have been an Indian rhino. Another mythical creature is the fire breathing dragon, a couple of which were featured in the recent TV epic series 'Game of Thrones'. This myth is likely to have arisen from religious medieval pictures depicting the entrance to hell that often showed a monster's literal mouth, with flames and smoke being emitted! These kinds of examples therefore illustrate how necessary it is to rely on a firm evidential basis before deducing the veracity of historical events.

Determining the age of past events

In order to find out what happened during the long history of the Earth we need to study its rocks scientifically and draw conclusions about the fossils that have been found embedded in them. If one can accurately determine the age of the rock, it follows that this will also be the age of the fossil found within it. Rocks can be of many different kinds. Their age determination and those of meteorites is carried out using sophisticated radiometric methods which measures how far certain radioactive elements contained within the rocks have decayed since their formation to produce stable by-product elements. By determining the ratio of stable by-product to original element in a sample of rock this will give an accurate age of that rock from its molten origin.

1. The Earth's formation and initial life

We need to establish a timeline and this starts with the formation of the solar system with the sun at its centre and nine orbiting planets which arose approximately 5 billion years ago:

https://www.nhm.ac.uk/discover/how-our-solar-system-was-born.html

Radiometric studies carried out on small crystals of Zircon from the Jack Hills of Western Australia have resulted in an age of 4.4 billion years old, while the age of the most ancient meteoritic material was found to be slightly older. In this way the age of the Earth in its initial likely molten state has been determined to be approximately 4.5 billion years old:

video: https://www.youtube.com/watch?v=oe45GegJUvM

After the Earth cooled down, its rocky surface formed, and the ages of seven of the most ancient rocks so far discovered have been found to be in the range of 3.8 – 4.2 billion years old.

http://www.oldest.org/geography/rocks/

The formation of our moon is considered to have been caused by an interaction of the still molten Earth with another large planetoid passing by which ejected a portion of its material:

https://www.nhm.ac.uk/discover/how-did-the-moon-form.html

The characterisation of life

A living creature can be defined by the following characteristics: they a) grow and change, b) reproduce to have offspring, c) have a complex chemistry, d) pass their traits on to their offspring, e) have a cellular structure, and f) respond to their environment.

The first lifeforms on Earth

These were the two types of microbial life that still exist today: **Bacteria** and **Archaea**. These are similar in appearance, but are distinguished by a number of characteristics:

1. Bacterial cell walls have a chemical called peptidoglycan (giving a mesh-like structure) while archaeal cell walls do not. Archaeal cell walls are structurally more diverse and contain more robust ether linkages (C-O-C) over those of bacteria, which gives them greater stability and protection from their environments.

2. Because of these cell wall differences, bacteria cannot live above 100 degrees Celsius; while archaea can thrive in a much broader range of chemical and temperature extremes. This has led them to being called **extremophiles**, since they are known to survive in extreme physical and geochemical conditions:

3. Bacterial growth is inhibited by antibiotics; but archaeal growth is not.

https://ucmp.berkeley.edu/archaea/archaea.html

Although bacteria and archaea are likely to have originated at about the same time during the early part of Earth's history, we will for the time being concentrate on ancient bacterial life and its impact upon the environment, before encountering archaea later when their vital importance to the establishing of higher lifeforms becomes apparent.

https://micro.magnet.fsu.edu/cells/bacteriacell.html

https://sciencing.com/nutritional-types-bacteria-2515.html

The evidence for ancient bacteria

The best example is fossilised microbial mats called Stromatolites that look like layered rocks and are found in Western Australia. These are estimated to be 3.5 billion years old.

https://newsroom.unsw.edu.au/news/science-tech/earliest-signs-life-scientists-find-microbial-remains-ancient-rocks

The microbes that usually inhabit these mats are specialised bacteria called cyanobacteria (also incorrectly known as 'blue-green algae' since they are NOT algae). They are special because they require water and sunlight to live. Hence the reason for the mats being found close to sea shores. Modern versions of these structures are visible today:

https://evolution.berkeley.edu/evolibrary/article/side_0_0/origsoflife_02

The way that bacteria 'live'

Normal bacteria do so by absorbing nutrients through their cell walls - but instead of growing in size they split into two (a process called Binary Fission). The resulting two cells will themselves split into two others to give a total of four, and so on, so that eventually a huge number of near-identical cells will result:

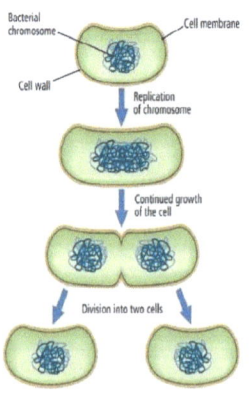

Binary Fission in Bacteria

Ref: https://www.goconqr.com/de-CH/p/4760948?dont_count=true&frame=true&fs=true

When it comes to the cyanobacteria, they don't simply rely on absorbing nutrients through their cell walls, but are adapted to absorb the gas carbon dioxide and react it with water to create sugars using the action of sunlight as an energy source. In this way they resemble the plants of today by employing the sun's energy and CO_2 to multiply. The reason why they were among the first bacteria to arise is that in the early Earth there was a plentiful amount of the CO_2 gas in the atmosphere - but no oxygen.

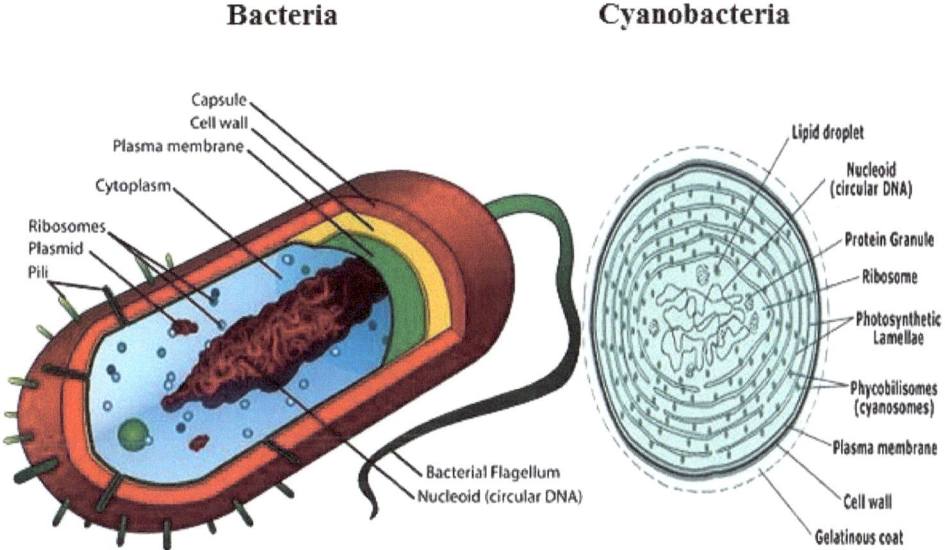

Ref: https://microbiologynotes.com/differences-between-bacteria-and-cyanobacteria/

The ability of bacteria to control their proliferation

The controlling factor of the splitting is the bacterial genome inside the cell which is made up of a long circular molecule called DNA. This molecule is the 'instruction manual' for all the processes that take place inside the cell - and is in fact the basis of all life on Earth. As the bacteria feeds through absorption there comes a point when this DNA molecule makes a copy of itself (i.e. replicates) to pass on to the daughter cell. It is this ability of the DNA molecule to replicate that enables all life on Earth to grow and multiply.

How does DNA replicate?

The DNA molecule exists in the form of a double helix made up of a pair of long sequences of four chemicals known as 'nitrogenous bases' named Adenine (A), Guanine (G), Thymine (T) and Cytosine (C). The two strands of the DNA each have a sugar-phosphate backbone and are loosely attached to one another by the base A coupling to T, and base G coupling to C. In order for replication to occur, the two strands uncouple and each strand is then built up with complimentary bases to form another one, so that one double helix gives rise to two of them (i.e. a 'replication' has occurred). It is unnecessary to know the chemical background of these compounds, but simply to think of them as the 'letters' A,T,G, and C that can be used in code form. For comparison, in the bacteria E. coli the circular DNA consists of 4 million base pairs, while that of human DNA consists of 3.1 billion base pairs!

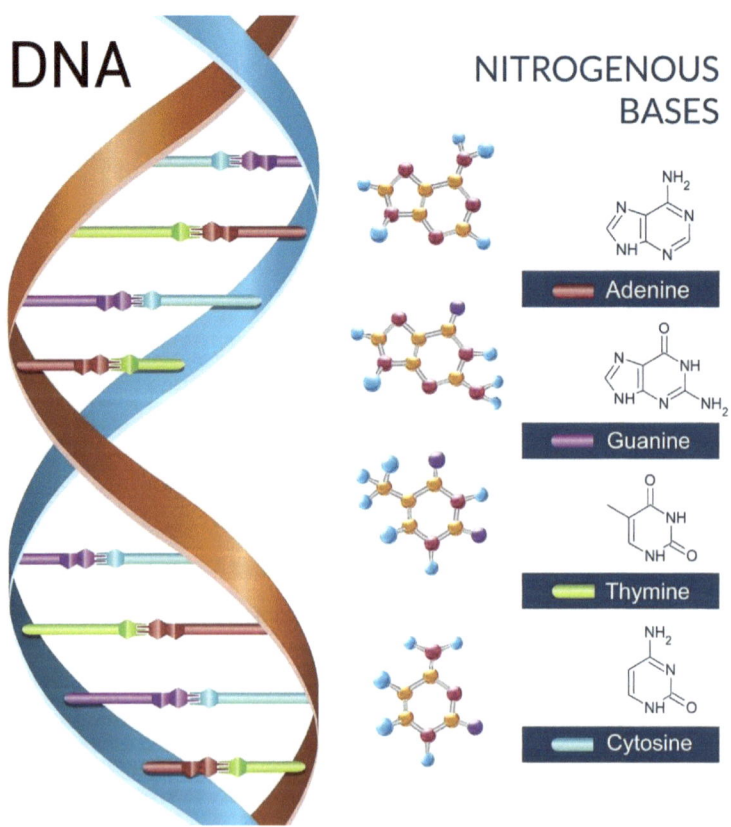

Ref: https://www.medicalnewstoday.com/articles/319818

What does the DNA do inside the cell?

It essentially provides coded instructions to construct large molecules from smaller ones. The four bases are similar to letters of an alphabet which can be 'read' in sequence in order for the cell to make the proteins that are vital for its existence. The latter are made up by linking together single amino acids in series, and there are a total of **twenty naturally occurring amino acids** to choose from.

https://www.chemistryworld.com/features/why-are-there-20-amino-acids/3009378.article?adredir=1

Each amino acid requires three of the bases to be read in sequence (which is called a DNA codon), and many of the amino acids are represented by more than one codon. For example, the amino acid Tryptophan has only one codon (TGG) while Serine has a total of six DNA codons that will enable it to be chosen for construction of a protein (also called a polypeptide).

Amino Acid	3 Letter Abbreviation	IUPAC Notation	Translating Codons
Alanine	Ala	A	GCT, GCC, GCA, GCG
Arginine	Arg	R	CGT, CGC, CGA, CGG, AGA, AGG
Asparagine	Asn	N	AAT, AAC
Aspartic acid	Asp	D	GAT, GAC
Cysteine	Cys	C	TGT, TGC
Glutamine	Gln	Q	CAA, CAG
Glutamic acid	Glu	E	GAA, GAG
Glycine	Gly	G	GGT, GGC, GGA, GGG
Histidine	His	H	CAT, CAC
Isolucine	Ile	I	ATT, ATC, ATA
Methionine	Met	M	ATG or START
Leucine	Leu	L	TTA, TTG, CTT, CTC, CTA, CTG
Lysine	Lys	K	AAA, AAG
Phenylalanine	Phe	F	TTT, TTC
Proline	Pro	P	CCT, CCC, CCA, CCG
Serine	Ser	S	TCT, TCC, TCA, TCG, AGT, AGC
Threonine	Thr	T	ACT, ACC, ACA, ACG
Tryptophan	Trp	W	TGG
Tyrosine	Tyr	Y	TAT, TAC
Valine	Val	V	GTT, GTC, GTA, GTG
STOP	Stop	*	TAA, TGA, TAG

So, let's take as an example a sequence of uncoiled DNA which has the following series of nitrogenous bases and is being 'read':

-Adenine-Thymine-Guanine-Thymine-Adenine-Thymine-Cytosine-Adenine-Thymine-Cytosine-Adenine-Adenine-Thymine-Thymine-Thymine-Guanine-Adenine-Thymine-Thymine-Guanine-Guanine-Thymine-Adenine-Guanine-

This can be represented in a short, three letter form as:

ATG-TAT-CAT-CAA-TTT-GAT-TGG-TAG

The first three letters would stand for the amino acid methionine if the sequence had already started, but if it's the first in line to be read it signifies a START signal. The next code TAT stands for the amino acid tyrosine which is then followed by CAT (= histidine) and then CAA (= glutamine), then TTT (= phenylalanine), then GAT, TGG (= aspartic acid, tryptophan) and lastly TAG which is a STOP signal. So the final series of linked amino acids produced would be:

Tyr-His-Gln-Phe-Asp-Trp

Since this structure is composed of only six amino acids it wouldn't be called a protein but rather a hexa-peptide - or - generically: a polypeptide. The largest protein in the human body is muscle tissue called Titin which is composed of 27,000 amino acids, while the smallest is Thyroid Releasing Hormone (TRH) which is made up of 234 amino acids. The smallest polypeptide in humans is Insulin which has 54 amino acids. Generally, a polypeptide needs to be larger than 100 amino acids for it to be called a protein.

How are the DNA codons read?

An enzyme called RNA polymerase partially unwinds the DNA molecule while building a complimentary molecule called **messenger RNA** (mRNA) having the equivalent sequence of codons for the protein synthesis. This is called the transcription phase. Once the mRNA has been built it is then transferred to the Ribosome within the cell where **ribosomal RNA** (rRNA) translates the information to make the protein molecule using the individual amino acids brought in separately by **transfer RNA** (tRNA).

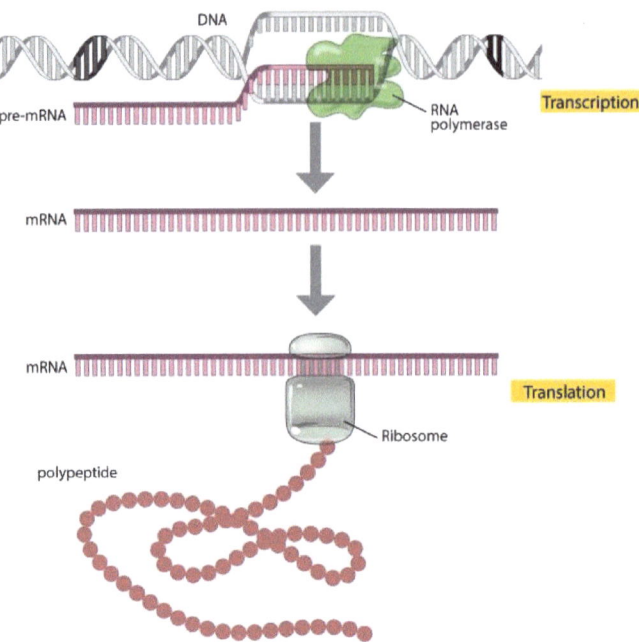

Ref: https://www.nature.com/scitable/topicpage/translation-dna-to-mrna-to-protein-393/

Video: https://www.youtube.com/watch?v=gG7uCskUOrA

RNA similarity to DNA

RNA molecules are very similar to that of a single strand of DNA, but are of shorter varying lengths and have subtle differences in the way that the sugar phosphate backbone contains ribose as the sugar molecule instead of deoxyribose, and also that the nitrogenous base

Thymine (T) is replaced by Uracil (U). This is why DNA is an abbreviation for **Deoxyribonucleic acid** while RNA is short for **Ribonucleic acid**. The 'acid' part of the name comes from the acidic phosphate groups that make up the backbone of each molecule:

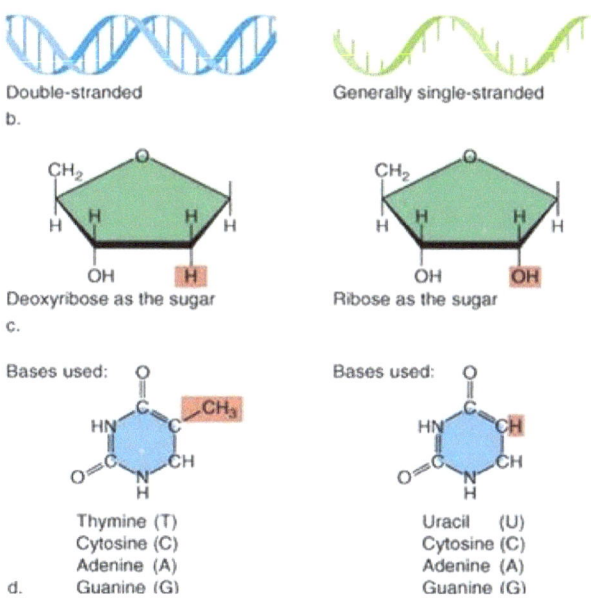

Ref: https://laboratoryinfo.com/dna-vs-rna/

How did the molecules DNA and RNA come into existence?

The clue lies in the fact that the two molecules are very similar, and while DNA serves as the master instruction code for defining a lifeform, the various RNA molecules involved are crucial in carrying out the tasks necessary for protein synthesis in order to achieve the lifeform's growth and development.

https://www.thoughtco.com/dna-versus-rna-608191

It is widely accepted by scientists that a pre-requisite for establishing life is the formation of a self-replicating molecule which could make copies of itself using chemicals from within the local environment. Chemical researchers in this field have therefore been working to confirm this by synthesizing similar compounds to establish that they can self-replicating with some good success. Because of such research the conclusion has been drawn that since RNA type molecules can both self-replicate and act as enzymes (i.e. as chemical catalysts) they were likely to have been the very first type of essential compounds that arose and eventually led to the emergence of bacterial life. Those investigating this outcome have called that period of time in Earth's early history as **'The RNA World'**.

Video: https://www.youtube.com/watch?v=K1xnYFCZ9Yg

https://www.newscientist.com/article/mg21128251-300-first-life-the-search-for-the-first-replicator/

https://www.newscientist.com/article/2088006-building-blocks-of-lifes-first-self-replicator-recreated-in-lab/

What happened next?

So, we have an early Earth on which the only primitive life present were bacteria and archaea. Most of these lived in an oxygen free environment and were therefore classified as anaerobic - i.e. their lives were not dependent upon oxygen. But this changed when the type of photosynthetic bacteria known as cyanobacteria mentioned earlier started to dominate, because their proliferation led to a change in the Earth's atmosphere! A by-product of photosynthesis is the gas oxygen which started to flow into the atmosphere. But oxygen is a very reactive element so it was initially absorbed by the abundant soluble iron salts contained within the oceans to generate an insoluble rust-like material which was deposited onto the sea beds. These deposits are found in many areas of the world and are called 'banded iron formations'.

Video: https://www.youtube.com/watch?v=E8-4IZGgfvY

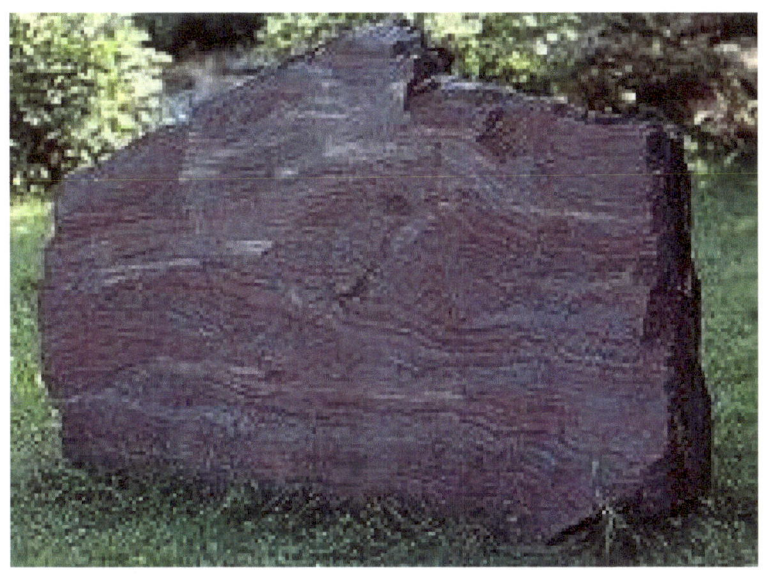

2.1-billion-year-old rock showing banded iron formation.

Ref: https://www.britannica.com/science/banded-iron-formation

These iron and other mineral depositions lasted for about a billion years before saturation of the oceans occurred and the oxygen then began to build up in the atmosphere. But even then the gas was also readily absorbed by the plentiful rocks situated on the land, so that it took another billion or so years before the proportion of oxygen in the atmosphere finally began to rise significantly from about 850 million years ago (**see below Stages 4 & 5**):

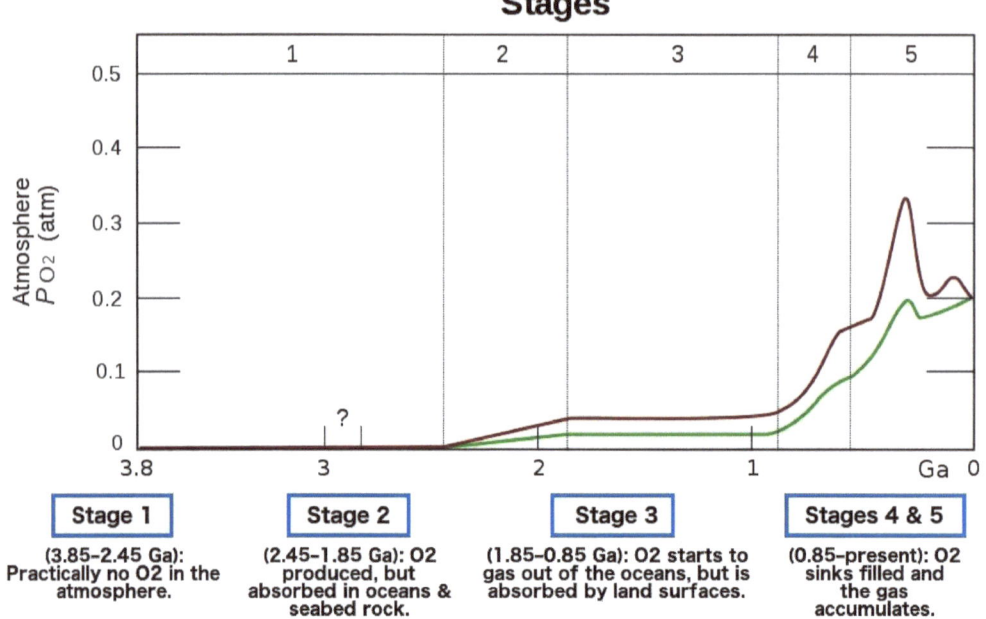

(The red vs green lines represent the range of estimates from different sources. Ga stands for Giga annum which is equivalent to one billion years).

Ref: https://www.ncbi.nlm.nih.gov/pmc/articles/PMC1578726/

The importance of this is evident because all complex life on Earth including ourselves depend upon the breathing in of oxygen for existence, so we can already appreciate that if it wasn't for the rise of cyanobacteria billions of years ago, we wouldn't be here!

What were the effects of oxygen build-up in the atmosphere?

The first thing that happened was the destruction of most of the anaerobic micro-organisms that were previously happy to live in an oxygen-free environment. The presence of oxygen had become poisonous for them. But the most important event that took place was the first appearance of unusual large sea-borne creatures called Ediacarans around 580 million years ago, signifying the initiation of complex lifeforms.

2. Complex life initiation

Ediacaran life was very crude in appearance and many appeared almost plant like, because they lacked anatomical features such as eyes or limbs, etc. One of the first fossils discovered in this group was from Charnwood Forest, Leicestershire in 1958 by a school boy named Roger Mason. The species - which resembled a fern - was called Charnia Masoni in recognition of his discovery.

https://www2.le.ac.uk/news/blog/2013/november/the-key-to-the-beginnings-of-life-on-earth-2013-found-by-a-schoolboy-in-charnwood-forest

http://www.ediacaran.org/charnwood-uk.html

https://www.astrobio.net/origin-and-evolution-of-life/fossils-on-the-edge-of-forever/

A much more recent fossil finding from this period was that of the oldest bilaterian creature (i.e. having a symmetric body) discovered in Australia which looked like a worm, and lived approximately 550 million years ago.

http://www.sci-news.com/paleontology/ikaria-wariootia-08254.html

The Cambrian Explosion

But the Ediacaran period didn't last long. Around 40 million years later a rapid mushrooming of complex lifeforms occurred in the oceans which also saw the demise of the Ediacarans and is called the Cambrian Explosion. The creatures that developed during this phase now took on appearances which are much more familiar to us by having eyes, a mouth and other anatomical features that commonly exist in the animal species of present today. A great number of shelly fossils have been found from this period showing that both prey and predator existed which may have been a strong factor in the diversity of life that arose during this period that lasted approximately 25 million years.

Video: https://www.youtube.com/watch?v=qNtQwUO9ff8

https://burgess-shale.rom.on.ca/en/science/origin/04-cambrian-explosion.php

Why did the proliferation of large creatures suddenly occur?

We know that the build-up of oxygen during that period was vital, because all complex life including humans that eventually followed need the intake of the oxygen for sustaining life. But to determine why this is the case we need to compare the cell structure of a typical animal with that of bacteria. One of the main differences is that complex lifeforms have in their cells a nucleus that contains **most** of their DNA, while bacteria and archaea do not. For this reason the former are called **Eukaryotes** (meaning cells **with a** nucleus) while the latter are named **Prokaryotes** (cells **without** a nucleus). The Eukaryotic cell also contains other components called organelles whose functions are unnecessary to discuss now, apart from one which is very important for our story, and that is the **mitochondrion**. As shown in the comparison sketch below, there are six mitochondria in the Eukaryotic half of the diagram, while there are none in the Prokaryotic half.

Comparison of Eukaryotic vs Prokaryotic cells

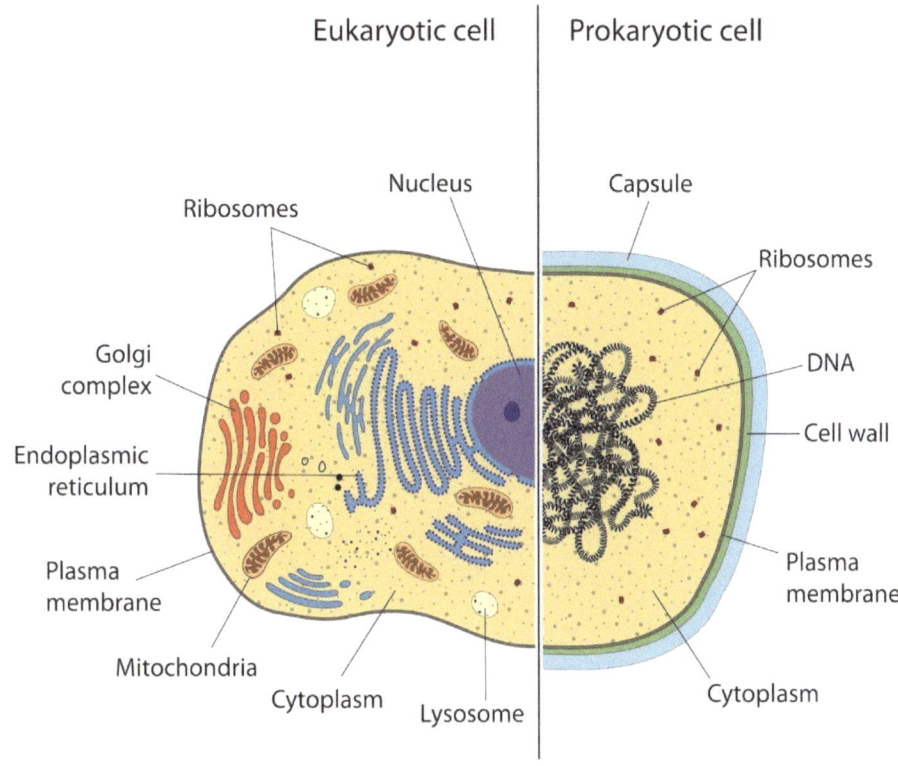

Ref: https://www.livescience.com/65922-prokaryotic-vs-eukaryotic-cells.html

The importance of the mitochondria lies in the fact that they provide energy for the cell. They act like little batteries, but instead of producing electrical energy as a battery would do, they provide a chemical version. In the human body any organ that is constantly active will be endowed with a great many mitochondria per individual cell. As an example, the human heart is an organ that works ceaselessly from birth to pump blood around the body. Each heart muscle cell contains around 5000 mitochondria to enable it to function continuously. In contrast, human liver cells that are not so physically active have between 1000-2000 mitochondria per cell. And for tiny human sperm to fertilize the egg in the female ovary they have to swim up the fallopian tube by whipping their tails to provide the necessary motion. The energy that's required to do this is supplied by 50-75 mitochondria situated just behind the head of each sperm.

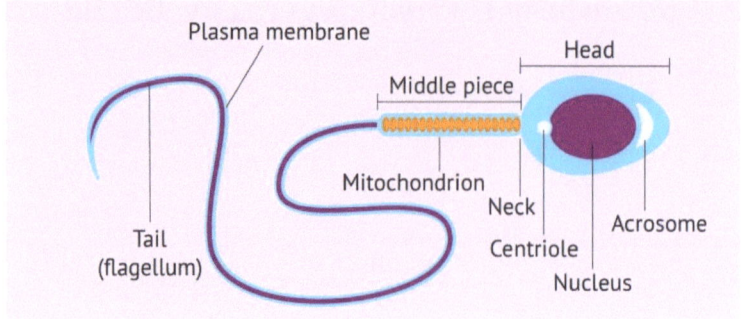

Ref: https://www.invitra.com/en/sperm-cell/

How is the chemical energy provided?

This is done through the supply of high-energy ATP molecules (adenosine triphosphate) which break down to release their energy as and when required by the cell. The ATP molecules are, in turn, produced by chemically 'burning' glucose (obtained from food) using oxygen (derived from aortal blood) within the mitochondria to afford the ATP along with CO_2 as a by-product. This is a process referred to as cellular respiration – but better known by name as the Krebs cycle or the tricarboxylic acid cycle.

The mitochondria enable large creatures to exist

By grouping together cells containing mitochondria it allows separate organs to form – such as the heart – to provide individual tasks for sustaining a complex lifeform. But they can only do this in the presence of oxygen gas. Animals breathe in this gas using their lungs in order to then 'burn' the food that they eat which enables the billions of mitochondria present in their bodies to furnish the energy that all their organs require to function normally. This is why large complex lifeforms **only became possible once oxygen levels arose significantly** during the Cambrian Explosion which started approximately 540 million years ago.

Where did the mitochondria come from?

If one investigates carefully the structure and activity of the mitochondria it becomes very apparent that they have a strong resemblance to bacterial cells! For example they have their own cell membranes, just like bacteria do, and also contain a circular spool of DNA within them – exactly like bacteria. They also make copies of themselves by binary fission – just as bacteria do. In 1967 the evolutionary biologist Lynn Margulis published a paper in the Journal of Theoretical Biology entitled 'On the Origin of Mitosing Cells' in which she proposed that the mitochondrion had once been a bacterial cell that had been engulfed by another, with the result that one bacterial cell lived inside another for their mutual benefit! Biologists were initially taken aback by this notion, but evidence soon accumulated from further research, which together with later genetic evidence, established beyond any doubt that this engulfing had indeed occurred in a process called **Endosymbiosis**. The surprising finding from the later genetic data was that the engulfing of a bacterial cell had not been done by another bacterium, but by its cousin the archaeon!

When and where did this engulfing event occur?

It is believed to have happened approximately 2 billion years ago, because the first examples of eukaryotic fossils in the form of microalgae were found in 1.5 billion year old rocks in northern Australia.

https://www.mpg.de/9256248/eukaryotes-evolution

Regarding where this might have happened, recent studies by Japanese researchers has revealed how it might have arisen on a deep-sea bed. Using a submersible craft they descended to recover mud samples from a 2500 meter deep ridge off the coast of Japan in 2006. These were incubated in bioreactors supplied with methane gas for over 5 years before isolating microbes which included an **Asgard species** of archaeon which was already known to have genetic similarities to eukaryotes. This microbe was then allowed to multiply – doubling in number during a period of 20 days instead of the usual 45 minutes or so for normal bacteria, after which they used an electron microscope to image one, which revealed tentacle-like appendages that could potentially reach out and drag other microbes within it. This method of trapping other microbes was actually predicted by the evolutionary biologist David Baum in 2014.

https://www.sciencemag.org/news/2019/08/tentacled-microbe-could-be-missing-link-between-simple-cells-and-complex-life

https://news.wisc.edu/new-theory-suggests-alternate-path-led-to-rise-of-the-eukaryotic-cell/

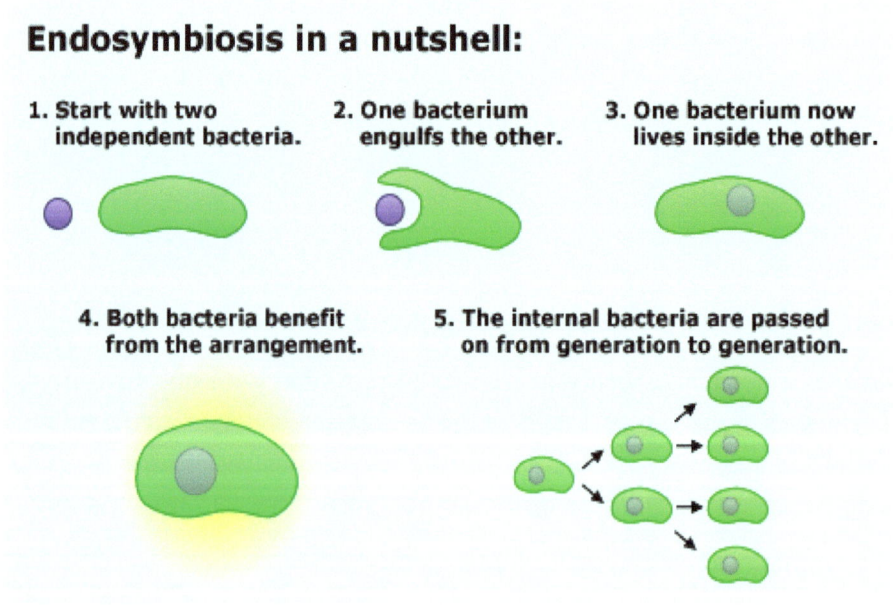

Ref: https://evolution.berkeley.edu/evolibrary/article/_0/endosymbiosis_03

Why did they look to find the archaeon on the sea bed?

The deep ocean is considered to be a primary candidate where microbial life could have started. Scientifically, it is widely accepted that for life to have been initiated using raw chemical ingredients there would have to have been a **continuous source of energy** from somewhere. This is because chemical reactions require energy to take place, and the complexity of even simple bacterial life would demand a whole series of such events to occur for it to have been produced. In 2000 a deep sea vent was discovered in the mid-Atlantic from which warm to hot alkaline fluids (45-90°C) containing dissolved minerals were seeping out from the ocean floor into the acidic sea water above. As the mixing of the two solutions took place it led to the formation of chimney-like insoluble carbonate structures 30-60m tall to be deposited. This first discovery was named The Lost City Hydrothermal Field although other similar alkaline vents have since been found elsewhere under the oceans. Because of their unique chemical environments these vents were found to harbour various types of microbial life inside or very close to them, in particular those of the Archaea extremophile type. These were able to live off the hydrogen and methane gases which also emanated from within the vents.

https://en.wikipedia.org/wiki/Lost_City_Hydrothermal_Field

Why are alkaline vents considered important for the initiation of life?

The alkaline solution exuding from the sea floor is usually hot (i.e. it has thermal energy to initiate reactions) but more importantly by introducing it into sea water which is naturally acidic (as derived from dissolved CO_2) the mixing promotes a gradient pH differential which is analogous to the (+) and (-) terminals of a battery. This particular environment is hypothesised to have been a key factor in establishing the similar pH differentials that exist across all living cell membranes, enabling them to function properly.

https://www.chemistryworld.com/features/hydrothermal-vents-and-the-origins-of-life/3007088.article?adredir=1

http://nick-lane.net/wp-content/uploads/2016/12/OriginOfLife.pdf

What type of bacterium was engulfed by the archaeon?

By comparing the genetic make-up of mitochondria with those of present day bacteria, the engulfed candidate is believed to have been a species of alphaproteobacteria which is known to be prevalent in sea water, although this identification is still subject to confirmation.

https://www.the-scientist.com/daily-news/mitochondrias-bacterial-origins-upended-33345

What happened after the engulfing of the bacterium?

The result was a cell with two sets of genes within it. Over time gene transfer occurred from the captured bacterium gene pool to the host archaeon genes to eventually result in a eukaryote type of cell. Once the Earth developed an oxygen atmosphere the smaller residual genetic component became a specialised organelle devoted to producing energy for the whole cell from the oxygen that was now available to it. This eventually led the eukaryotic cells to clump together and form simple animals that could evolve into larger ones.

https://www.nature.com/scitable/topicpage/the-origin-of-mitochondria-14232356/#

How did plants form?

These arose from a eukaryotic cell that additionally took inside (i.e. via a **second** endosymbiosis) another bacterial cell which was a photosynthetic cyanobacterium. This similarly transformed into an organelle called a **chloroplast** which enabled the eukaryotic cell to harvest energy from sunlight and eventually lead to the formation of large plants as revealed below:

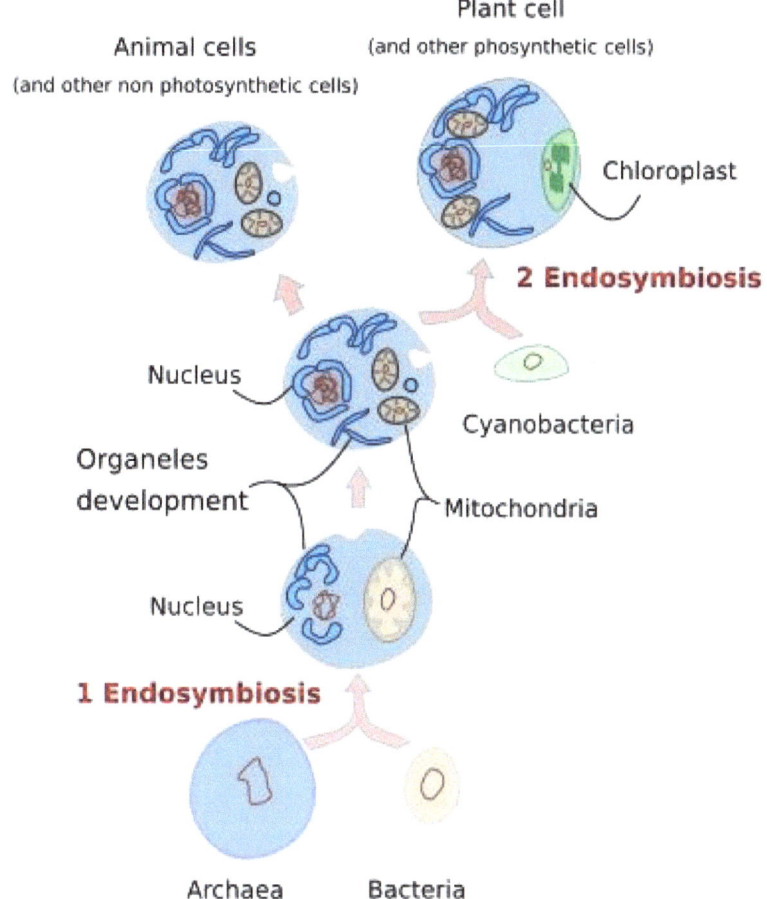

Ref: https://mmegias.webs.uvigo.es/02-english/5-celulas/1-endosimbiosis.php

A genetic analysis of a freshwater blue-green algae called glaucophyte - one of a small group known as "living fossils" - has revealed further information about how the very first plant might have been formed.

https://www.scientificamerican.com/article/how-first-plant-evolved/

So can we now imagine a 'tree of life'?

Yes, it is very clear from genetic evidence that the simple prokaryotes bacteria and archaea were initially formed approximately 3.8 billion years ago and that the first eukaryotes of which plants and animals are members originated between 1.6 and 2 billion years ago. Because the latter evolved from an archaeon the tree of life can be represented by the following three domains in which the eukaryota branch is an offshoot of the original archaea one:

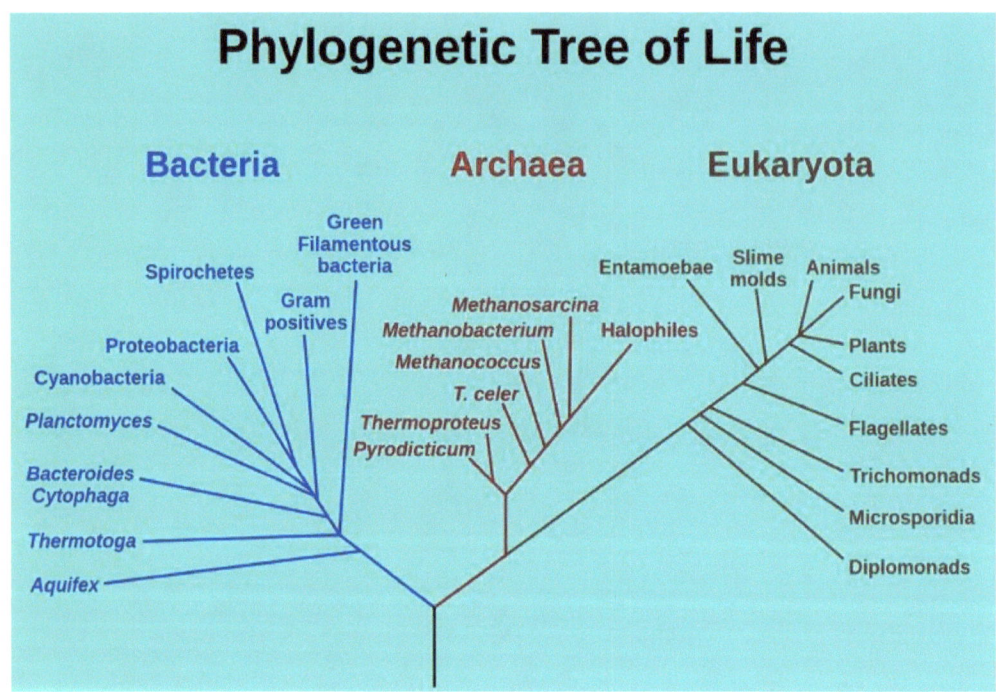

Ref: https://www.thoughtco.com/three-domain-system-373413

https://bio.libretexts.org/Bookshelves/Introductory_and_General_Biology/Book%3A_Introductory_Biology_(CK-12)/5%3A_Evolution/5.5%3A_Evolution_of_Eukaryotes

3. The evolutionary process

All lifeforms are able to change incrementally with time due to environmental constraints that favour one version over another. This slow process is known as **evolution through natural selection** and was first proposed by Darwin in his book '*The Origin of the Species*' published in 1860. The bottom part of the Tree of Life diagram above shows that all life emerged from a single source which was likely to have been a self-replicating RNA-type of molecule. This led to a primitive pre-bacterial cell which then diverged in two different paths to afford the first bacterial and archaeal lineages. Each of these further branched out to furnish the nine bacterial species and seven archaeal ones shown in the illustration. The evolution of one type of bacterium to result in several different ones has occurred because localised environmental conditions forced genomic changes to occur to allow for continued existence. As a current example we know that an infection caused by harmful bacteria can be treated with antibiotics to kill them, but if the treatment is not totally successful the small number remaining can then acquire immunity to the antibiotic and render it useless. This is classed as an evolutionary step for the bacterium.

An excellent example of the ability of forcing environmental factors to create a bewildering array of sub groups from a single species is the evolution of dogs from the Grey Wolf that occurred thousands of years ago. As early humans created dwellings to live in, they befriended amenable Grey Wolves as pets as well as for security reasons, just as people do today with dogs. Eventually, depending upon the type of treatment these wolves were subjected to during domestication, they slowly morphed into creatures more suited to their new living conditions. Further cross breeding by humans to confer favourable attributes such as shortness, strength, stub nose, etc. led to the huge number of dog varieties that exist today.

Video: https://www.youtube.com/watch?v=nDt0HKSdRRw

https://web.archive.org/web/20120301134035/http://www.provet.co.uk/dogs/evolution%20of%20the%20dog.htm

There are many other examples of evolution that are of more recent origin.

https://phys.org/news/2018-11-human-evolution-possibly-faster.html

http://www.bbc.co.uk/earth/story/20150803-how-do-we-know-evolution-is-real

What are the simplest examples of Eukaryotes living today?

The most obvious are single cell organisms called Protists, examples of which are amoebas, algae and ciliates. Their ancestors would undoubtedly have been present at the dawn of the eukaryotic period nearly 2 billion years ago. Although they all have mitochondria for energy production purposes, some have specialised versions which do not rely on oxygen for respiration and are therefore found in anoxic conditions. A pertinent example is the sexually transmitted parasite *Trichomonas vaginalis*, which infects the human vagina and causes **problems**. In this instance the mitochondrion has been adapted to produce the necessary energy rich molecules of ATP as described earlier, but with concomitant generation of hydrogen as a side product, and for this reason the organelle is classified as a hydrogenosome.

What is surprising is that even though amoebas are small and rather simple creatures they have been found to have the **largest genomes known among eukaryotes**, with the 'dubia-amoeba' variety having 670 billion units of DNA, which is over 200 times larger than that of humans!

http://www.genomenewsnetwork.org/articles/02_01/Sizing_genomes.shtml

Another simple eukaryote is the lancelet which has a very basic animal structure comprising of a simple head, body and tail. This creature lives in shallow sandy areas of seas around the world which they inhabit by embedding their bodies into the sand and filter-feeding on plankton from their head ends. This is an example of a 'living fossil' because Lancelets closely resemble 530-million-year-old *Pikaia*, which are known from ancient fossil bearing Burgess Shale in Canada.

https://ucmp.berkeley.edu/cambrian/burgess.html

They still contain a notochord running along the length of their body which is a very primitive version of the vertebrate that developed later in fishes and animals.

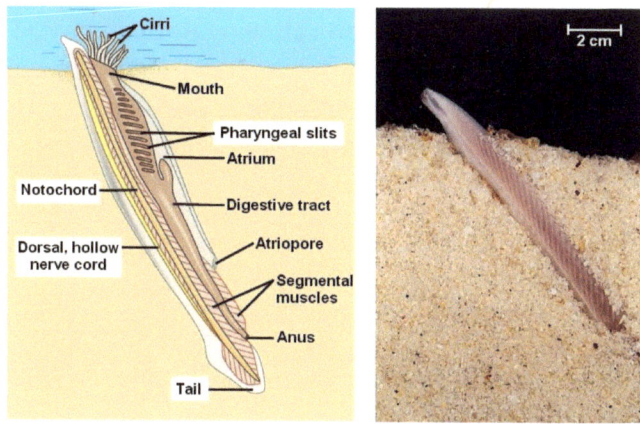

Ref: http://www.sliderbase.com/images/referats/1470b/(11).PNG

The lancelet is a modern example of a cephalochordate whose early evolutionary relevance to later vertebrates is shown below:

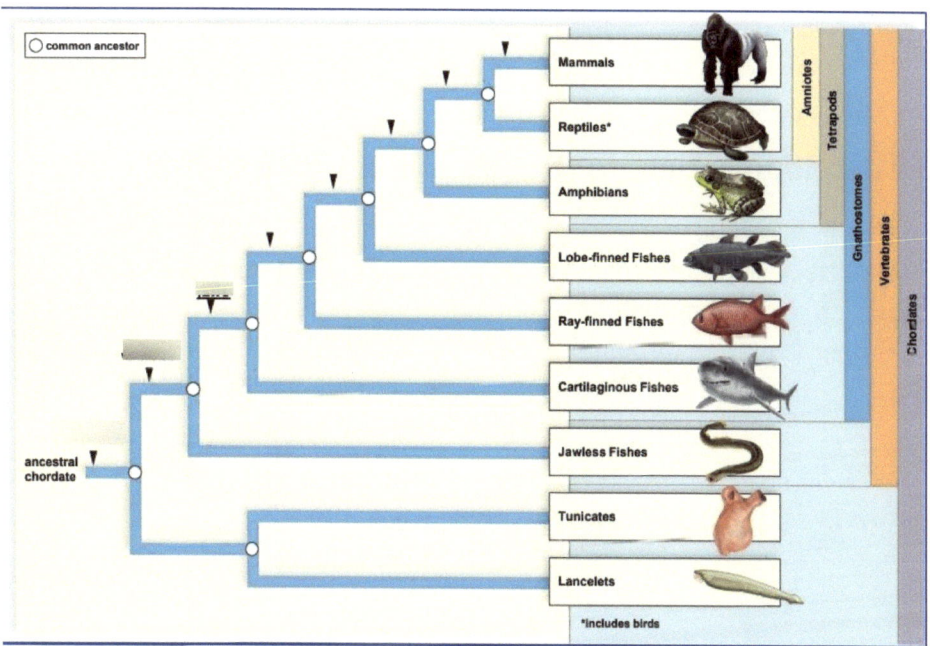

Ref: https://quizlet.com/273692575/phylogenetic-tree-of-the-chordates-diagram/

Video: Chordates: https://www.youtube.com/watch?v=kgZRZmEc9j4

Another example of a simple animal living today is the sea sponge which is normally found attached to submerged rocks while feeding on tiny creatures such as plankton derived from the water flowing through its body pores. Because of its very primitive multi-cellular structure it was considered to be one of the first types of animal that existed in evolutionary terms, but recent studies point to the comb jelly as a more likely candidate from genetic analysis.

https://animalsake.com/sponges-characteristics

https://cosmosmagazine.com/biology/the-first-animals-were-comb-jellies-genetic-study-finds

The Oxford University Museum of Natural History has recently had an exhibition on First Animals:

http://www.oum.ox.ac.uk/firstanimals/#group-First-Animals-iDULiuWNAB

The development of life after the Cambrian Explosion

The Cambrian Explosion formed the first part of the Paleozoic (meaning 'ancient life') Era, after which five others followed - starting with the Ordovician and ending with the Permian, a total period of 300 million years. The further evolution of plants and animals during this time is summarised below.

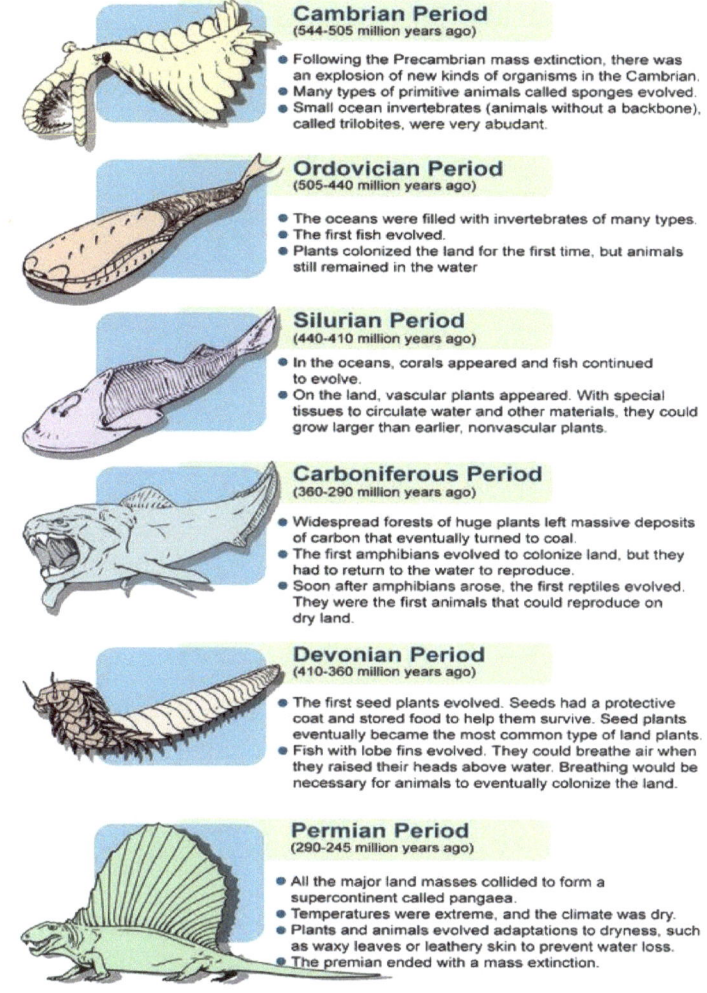

Ref: https://www.ck12.org/c/biology/paleozoic-era/lesson/Ancient-Plants-and-Animals-Advanced-BIO-ADV/

https://www.fossils-facts-and-finds.com/paleozoic_era.html

https://www.pbs.org/wgbh/evolution/change/deeptime/paleoz.html

Following the Paleozoic came the Mesozoic (meaning 'middle life') Era which was the age of the dinosaurs and encompassed the Triassic, Jurassic and Cretaceous periods, a total period of 180 million years. The following shows the continental groupings of the Earth during the Triassic period.

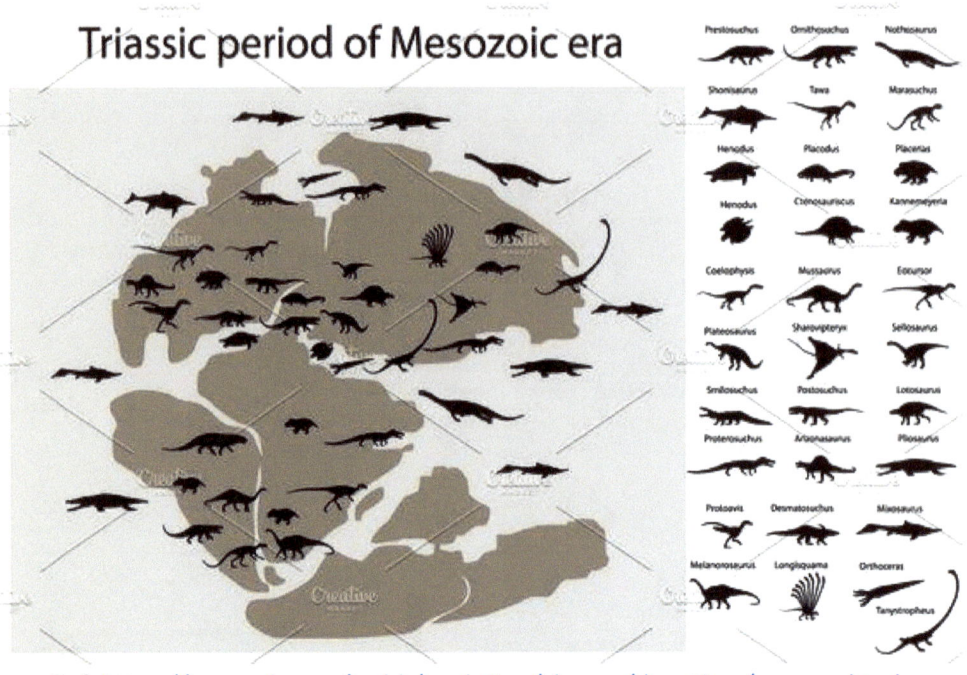

Ref: https://www.pbs.org/wgbh/evolution/change/deeptime/mesozo.html

Finally we come to the Cenozoic (meaning 'new life') Era, which is made up of the Paleocene, Eocene, Oligocene, Miocene, Pliocene, Pleistocene (ice age) and Holocene Epochs, a total of 65 million years to reach to the present day. The three Eras combined (540 million years) are called the Phanerozoic Eon.

Eon	Era	Period		Epoch	Start Date (mya)
Phanerozoic	Cenozoic	Quaternary		Holocene	0.01
				Pleistocene	1.64
		Tertiary	Neogene	Pliocene	5.2
				Miocene	23.3
			Paleogene	Oligocene	35.4
				Eocene	56.5
				Paleocene	65

Ref: https://hoopermuseum.carleton.ca/evolution/equidae/cenozoicera.html

https://www.pbs.org/wgbh/evolution/change/deeptime/cenozo.html

The entire geological history of the Earth can be summarised by the following diagram:

Geological Time Scale

ERA	PERIOD	EPOCH / AGE	Million Years Ago	EVENTS
CENOZOIC *Age of Mammals* 65.5 mya – present day	Quaternary	Holocene	Today – 0.01	Ice Age ends. Humans are dominant
		Pleistocene	0.01 – 1.6	Earliest Humans appear. Ice Age begins
	Tertiary	Pliocene	1.6 – 5.3	Hominids (human ancestors) appear
		Miocene	5.3 – 23.7	Grass becomes widespread
		Oligocene	23.7 – 36.6	Mammals are dominant
		Eocene	36.6 – 57.8	Eocene – Oligocene extinction event
		Paleocene	57.8 – 65.5	First large mammals appear
MESOZOIC *Age of Reptiles* 245 mya – 65.5 mya	Cretaceous	Extinction of Dinosaurs	65.5 – 144	K-T extinction event. Earth looks closer to present-day. Flowering plants appear
	Jurassic		144 – 208	First Birds appear. Pangaea splits into Laurasia, Gondwanna. Dinosaurs are dominant
	Triassic	First Dinosaurs	208 – 245	Pangaea cracks. First mammals appear. Reptiles are dominant
PALEOZOIC 570 mya – 245 mya	Permian	Age of Amphibians	245 – 286	Permian – Triassic extinction event. Pangaea forms
	Carboniferous		286 – 360	First reptiles appear. First large cartilaginous fishes appear
	Devonian	Age of Fishes	360 – 408	Late Devonian extinction event. First land animals appear. First amphibians appear
	Silurian		408 – 438	First land plants appear. First jawed fishes appear. First insects appear
	Ordovician	Age of Invertebrates	438 – 505	Ordovician – Silurian extinction event. First vertebrates appear
	Cambrian		505 – 570	End Botomian extinction event. First fungi appear. Trilobites are dominant
PRECAMBRIAN 4600 mya – 570 mya	Proterozoic Eon		570 – 2500	First soft-bodied animals appear. First multicellular life appear
	Achean Eon		2500 – 3800	Photosynthesizing cyanobacteria appear. First unicellular life appear
	Hadean Eon	Priscoan Period	3800 – 4600	Atmosphere and oceans form. Oldest rocks form as Earth cools

Formation of Earth

Ref: https://www.deviantart.com/andyckh/art/Geological-Timeline-Chart-283922560

Mass extinction events

By analysing rock strata carefully one can obtain evidence of at least five mass extinctions that occurred throughout Earth's history. This can be determined because an older rock layer containing many fossils may then be overlaid with a newer one containing far fewer, while there might also be an obvious change in the colour or mineral type for the two layers. The change could therefore be linked to volcanic activity or some other environmental catastrophe that lead to the extinction.

The five periods in which these occurred are 440, 375, 250, 200 and 65 million years ago, the last of which destroyed the dinosaurs.

https://www.thoughtco.com/the-5-major-mass-extinctions-4018102

The rise of the mammals

The last of the Eras - the Cenozoic - is the most important for ourselves because the demise of the dinosaurs at its beginning helped another group of animals - the mammals - to become dominant thereafter. There is strong evidence that the dinosaurs - which had existed for 165 million years - were killed off in a geological instant by a catastrophe caused by a 10 mile wide asteroid impacting the edge of the Yucatan peninsula in Mexico 65 million years ago. It is estimated that nearly 75% of all living species were eliminated from the firestorm that ensued. This event (also known as the **Cretaceous–Tertiary (K–T) or Cretaceous–Paleogene (K-Pg) extinction**) meant that the small number of mammals that ultimately survived could flourish free from predation by much larger creatures. Recent fossil recoveries have revealed that the earliest mammals co-existed with dinosaurs approximately 190 million years ago, but the main propagation occurred once the dinosaurs had disappeared.

https://phys.org/news/2019-06-mammals-relatives-diversified-so-called-age.html

https://www.nhm.ac.uk/discover/how-an-asteroid-caused-extinction-of-dinosaurs.html

What's special about mammals?

Mammals have four unique characteristics, the first two of which are related. They are:

      A) mammary glands
      B) sweat glands
      C) hair
      D) middle ear bones

https://www.thoughtco.com/the-main-mammal-characteristics-4086144

Fossil evidence shows that the early mammals were small shrew-like creatures which developed fur to keep themselves warm during cold weather, as well as to provide protection and camouflage from predators. Sweat glands developed mainly to keep them cool during warm weather or when expending energy through running, etc. But some sweat glands also became specialised to provide milk to their suckling young. In terms of giving birth, mammals can be grouped into three types (or phylogeny) starting with the most ancient in evolutionary terms: egg laying Monotremes such as the platypus (a relic from the dinosaur era), followed by pouch bearing Marsupials such as the kangaroo, and finally placental Eutherians such as humans and mice. The provision of milk to their young also differs:

https://www.britannica.com/science/mammary-gland

https://www.livescience.com/7488-world-strangest-creature-part-mammal-part-reptile.html

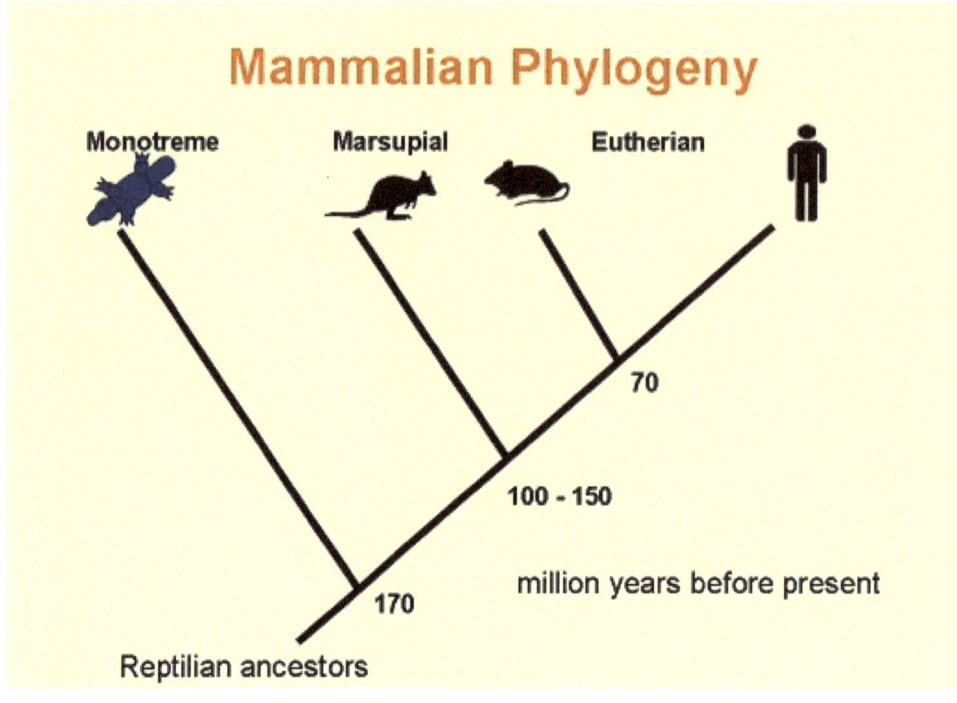

Ref: https://renfreeshawlab.biosciences.uom.org.au/resources/marsupials-an-introduction/

The evolution of the Great Apes

Of the 5000 species of mammal that exists today, the most relevant for us is the presence of approximately 300 species of the tree dwelling primates. If you flex your hands you can see how well they are constructed to firmly grip something like the branch of a tree. This dexterity is not an accident - it arises because our ancestors once lived an arboreal life on top of trees, just like most of our primate cousins still do to this day. The earliest primate from fossil evidence was a tree dwelling small nocturnal insect eater called Purgatorius which existed just after the demise of the dinosaurs. It is very similar to a tree shrew which is the closest living relative to primates today. Indeed, tree shrews are considered to be 'living fossils' of ancestral primates. The photo of the tree shrew below shows how it has the familiar four fingers and a thumb on each 'hand' along with similar five digits for their feet revealing their closeness to primates. The brains of these creatures are also more highly developed than those of mice for example, displaying the folded nature more characteristic of the brains of primates.

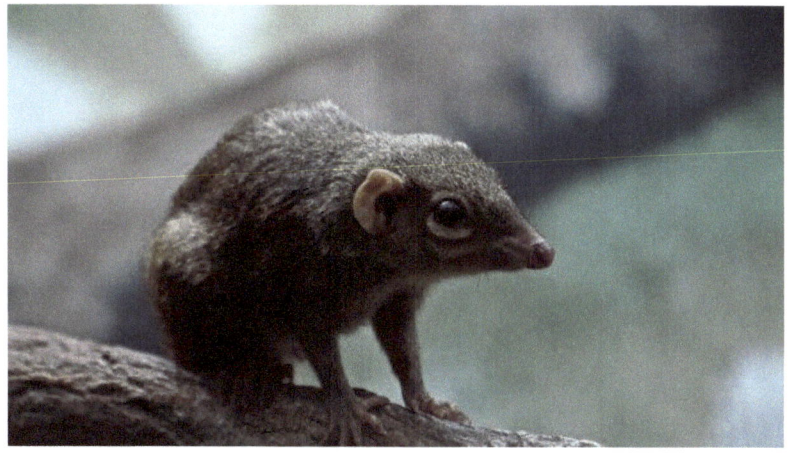

Ref: https://blogs.biomedcentral.com/on-biology/2017/12/18/ever-wondered-what-goes-on-in-a-tree-shrews-mind/

https://www.nationalgeographic.com/news/2012/10/121024-purgatorius-earliest-primate-evolution-science-squirrel/

The diagram below shows how the many types of primates that exist today descended from their ancestral primate likely to have been Purgatorius or a very similar creature.

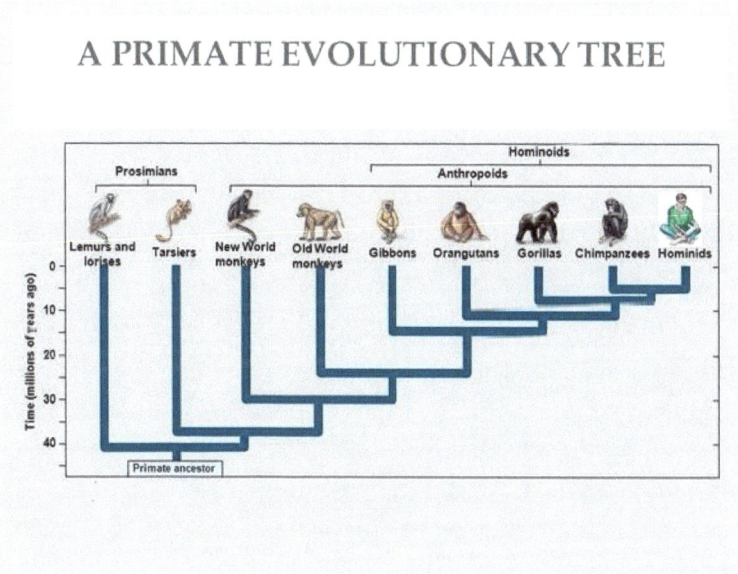

Ref: https://www.quora.com/If-you-are-now-to-the-apes-what-our-descendants-will-be-to-us-what-do-you-think-our-descendants-will-be-like

As the descendants of the tree shrews developed and grew into larger creatures they also consumed the leaves and fruits that the trees provided for sustenance, but these couldn't provide much in the way of protein. Our close cousins the chimps eventually turned to hunting other primates to acquire a more nutritious meat diet, which meant they had to spend more time on the ground foraging for food, as did the primate ancestors of humans.

https://www.theatlantic.com/science/archive/2016/02/when-humans-became-meateaters/463305/

https://www.nationalgeographic.co.uk/animals/2018/04/chimps-eat-baby-monkey-brains-first-clue-human-evolution

https://www.nature.com/scitable/knowledge/library/overview-of-hominin-evolution-89010983/

How did humans evolve?

This process started approximately 6 million years ago when our most ancient ancestral line diverged from one that led to present day chimpanzees. The cause will have been different environmental pressures acting on each, just like the ones that led to the present great variety of dogs that evolved from their ancient wolf ancestor. It should be noted that chimpanzees are categorized as apes not only because of their appearance but also because they use all four limbs to move around in the form of 'knuckle-walking'. In contrast, the early humans (called hominins) were already beginning to walk in an upright mode using just their feet.

In archaeological terms the most significant discovery occurred in the Afar region of Ethiopia in 1974 when the skeleton of a young female measuring 1.05 metres tall was found. This was nicknamed 'Lucy' because the discoverers often played the Beatles' song "Lucy in the Sky with Diamonds" during their leisure time. As would be expected, inspection of the skeleton revealed a mixture of human and ape like features, as well as showing that she had possibly died from injuries received from falling off a tree. Her fossil age was determined to be approximately 3.2 million years old by potassium-argon radiometric dating of the lava ash deposits that were above and below the rock layer that the skeleton was recovered from. She is a member of the ***Australopithecus afarensis*** hominin group (meaning southern ape from the Afar region) which as a species is estimated to have lasted for 700,000 years as evidenced from other similar fossils discovered. To put that into context, our present ***Home sapiens*** group has been around for only 200,000 years.

https://www.thoughtco.com/potassium-argon-dating-methods-1440803

https://iho.asu.edu/about/lucys-story

https://www.nhm.ac.uk/discover/australopithecus-afarensis-lucy-species.html

Over the last 50 years or so approximately 20 hominin types have been identified from their skeletal remains recovered mainly from the African continent. The closest one to humans in terms of appearance and walking gait was ***Home erectus*** which first appeared 1.9 million years ago and lasted until about 100,000 years ago. Its importance to us is that this was the likely species that left Africa thousands of years ago eventually leading directly to ***Homo Sapiens*** as well as its close cousin ***Homo Neanderthalensis*** that lived in Europe until about 40,000 years ago. Yet another close cousin is the ***Denisovan*** hominin, fragments of which were originally discovered 10 years ago inside a cave in Siberia. This appears from DNA evidence to be a sister group of Neanderthals but unfortunately there have been very few skeletal fragments so far identified.

http://humanorigins.si.edu/evidence/human-fossils/species/homo-erectus

https://www.nhm.ac.uk/discover/homo-erectus-our-ancient-ancestor.html

https://www.nhm.ac.uk/discover/who-were-the-neanderthals.html

https://www.nature.com/articles/d41586-019-02820-0

Video (Denisovans): https://www.youtube.com/watch?v=ytktpNIN3OM

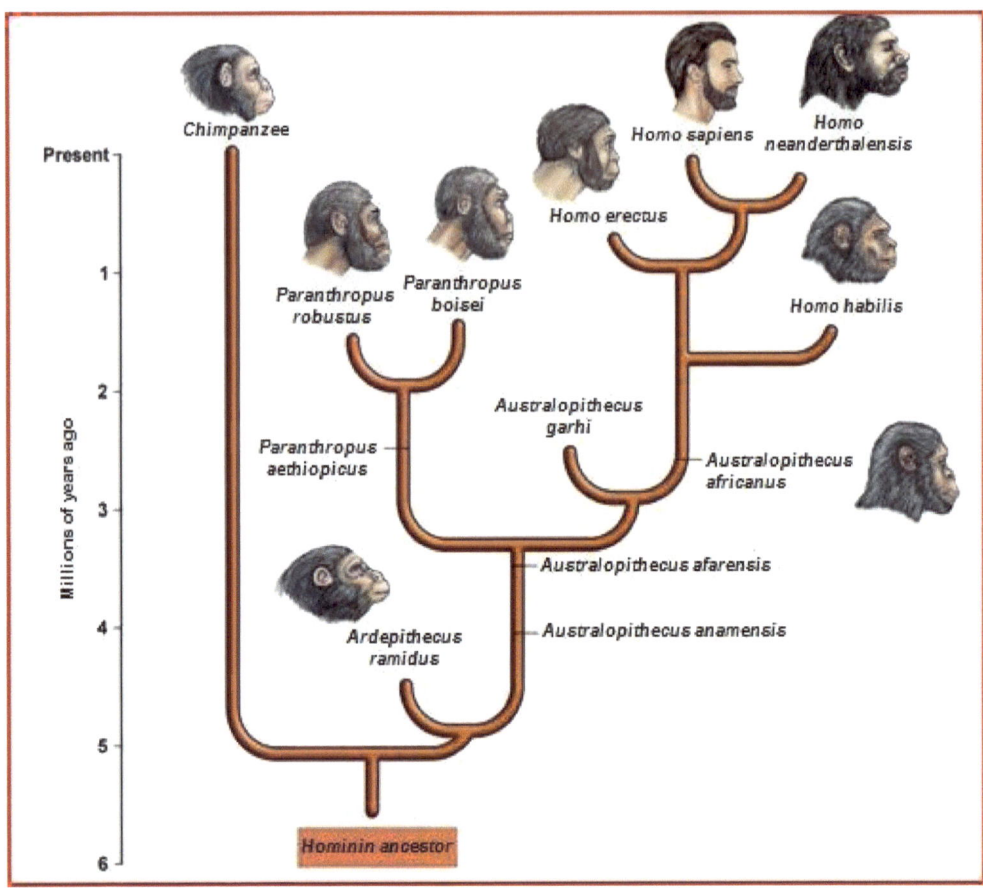

Ref: http://humanevolutionofficial.weebly.com/#PhotoSwipe1416814376779

An informative timeline for human evolution can be found here:

https://www.oxfordreference.com/view/10.1093/acref/9780191735349.timeline.0001

What are the main differences that distinguish humans from apes?

The genetic evidence for our close connection to the Great Apes is substantial - we all have a genomic equivalence greater than 98%! In contrast, all humans have a 99.9% similarity to each other, with the remaining 0.1% accounting for the variability in human appearances and characteristics.

Although the chimpanzee is often reported to be our closest ape relative, a recent study has established that bonobos are actually closer by reference to their muscle structures.

https://gwtoday.gwu.edu/bonobos-may-resemble-humans-more-you-think

One unique difference is that the human genome is distributed in 46 chromosomes as 23 pairs, while those of the apes all have 48 chromosomes as 24 pairs. From genetic investigations it has been determined that this change was caused by a fusion of a pair of ape chromosomes approximately 1-4 million years ago to result in an extended Chromosome No.2 for humans. It is probable that this fusion would have acted as an efficient reproductive wall that isolated us from the ancestors of the large apes.

https://www.bbvaopenmind.com/en/science/bioscience/the-origin-of-the-human-species-a-chromosome-fusion/

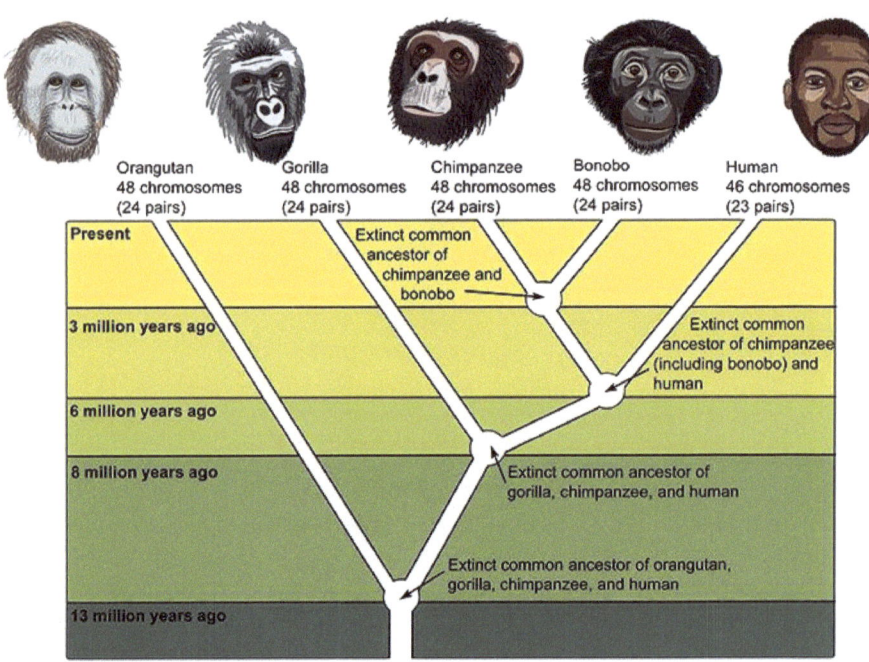

Ref: https://mammothmemory.net/biology/characteristics-and-classifications/classification/phylogenic-tree.html

Another notable difference is the relatively hairless nature of human skin. This is considered to have resulted once upright humans began to chase after animal prey with sharp weapons and needed to sweat to cool down. Having any kind of thick hair would have made this difficult and it was therefore slowly lost in response to the necessity of keeping cool while active.

http://www.bbc.co.uk/earth/story/20160801-our-weird-lack-of-hair-may-be-the-key-to-our-success

When it comes to intelligence humans are clearly on top of the group as far as mammals are concerned with their relatively large brain size being a strong determinate. By comparison chimps have a brain which is only one third the size of those of humans. But another factor is the greater degree of folding of the human brain which enables us to learn more quickly than chimps do. As mentioned with reference to sweating, early upright humans began to chase after animals in order to consume meat rich in protein, which will also have contributed to their greater brain enlargement starting from about 2.6 million years ago. And some researchers suggest that modern humans might never have appeared if the cooking of meat to release more easily digestible proteins to nourish their brains hadn't been discovered.

https://www.sciencemag.org/news/2015/11/humans-can-outlearn-chimps-thanks-more-flexible-brain-genetics

https://www.nature.com/scitable/knowledge/library/evidence-for-meat-eating-by-early-humans-103874273/

https://www.scientificamerican.com/article/food-for-thought-was-cooking-a-pivotal-step-in-human-evolution/

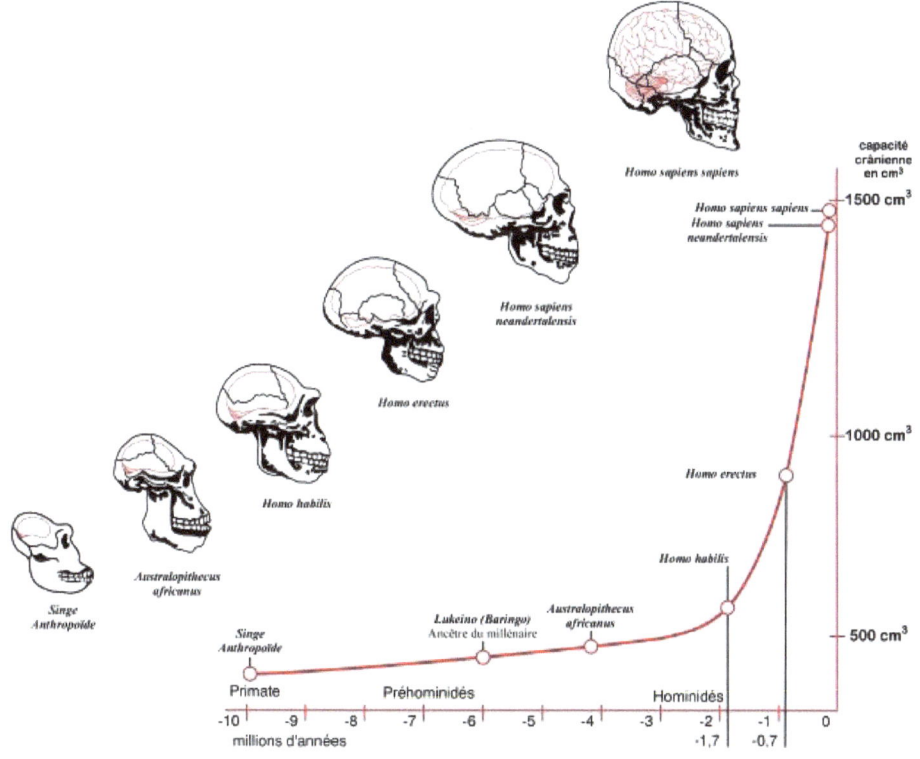

Growth of hominin brain capacity with time

Ref: https://www.filthymonkeymen.com/2011/12/25/explaining-our-big-brains/

Why do living things grow old and die?

We have seen how complex life including humans could only have arisen because of the presence of mitochondria producing energy for their organs by chemically 'burning' food using the oxygen they breathe in. Unfortunately, there is a downside to needing oxygen and that is the element's propensity to form **reactive free radicals** (i.e. by the loss of an electron) which can then cause serious damage to organs and tissues over a long period of time. Humans have a certain degree of protection from this by having enzymes such as superoxide dismutase to remove them. Further protection can also be gained through the ingestion of known anti-oxidant foods such as fruits and nuts as well as doing exercise.

https://www.psychologytoday.com/gb/blog/the-art-and-science-aging-well/201805/how-free-radicals-oxygen-accelerate-our-aging

Another factor that controls aging lies in a genetic 'clock' in the form of telomeres which protects DNA by being situated at the ends of chromosomes analogous to the hardened tips that protect the ends of shoe laces. Every time the cell divides this protective telomere shortens until eventually it's too short to be useful and the cell then becomes senescent and can no longer function properly. Experiments with mice have shown that killing these deleterious senescent cells can rejuvenate the younger cells that lie beneath.

https://www.the-scientist.com/features/can-destroying-senescent-cells-treat-age-related-disease--67136

https://www.sciencedaily.com/releases/2018/02/180227142114.htm

https://www.scientificamerican.com/article/to-stay-young-kill-zombie-cells/

https://www.varsity.co.uk/science/18066

https://www.sciencedaily.com/releases/2018/02/180227142114.htm

https://www.healthline.com/health/beauty-skin-care/premature-aging#signs-to-watch-for

https://news.harvard.edu/gazette/story/2019/03/anti-aging-research-prime-time-for-an-impact-on-the-globe/

4. The human genome and its quirks

We noted at the start of this book that the genome of a lifeform is a very long molecule called DNA containing 3-base codons which refer to particular amino-acids (out of 20 in total) that are read in sequence to enable the construction of a whole string of linked amino acids that's known as a polypeptide or protein depending upon its size. Such proteins will usually have a vital catalytic role to play in sustaining the lifeform's existence. The genetic code for that particular protein is called its 'gene'.

In humans the genome contains approximately 35,000 genes necessary for protein production, but this only represents less than 5% of the entire genome which contains 3.1 billion base pairs. Most of the remaining 95% has hitherto been described as 'junk' DNA in the past, but it is now known that at least 10-20% is considered vital in controlling many processes which is a field that is being vigorously investigated.

The genome normally exists as long strands called chromatin which are spooled around histone proteins within the cell's nucleus. When the cell prepares to divide these groupings condense to form the 23 paired chromosomes (i.e. one from each parent) which can be seen under a powerful microscope if suitably stained with a dye. One of these pairs (no.23) is called the sex chromosome, having either two X ones to confer the female sex, or a XY to confer the male sex, the Y coming from the male parent, and taking this distinction into account the other 22 pairs of chromosomes are then called Autosomes.

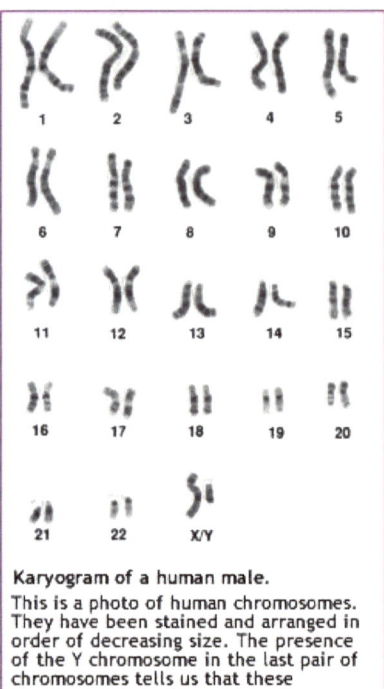

Ref: https://www.ncbi.nlm.nih.gov/books/NBK22266/

Following the condensation all 23 pairs are then duplicated, going through X-shaped 'sister chromatids' connected by the 'centromere' in the middle before the cell splits to give two daughter cells equivalent to the one existing before. This is done through a binary fission process (mitosis) in which spindle fibres attach to the centromere and pull the sister chromatids apart.

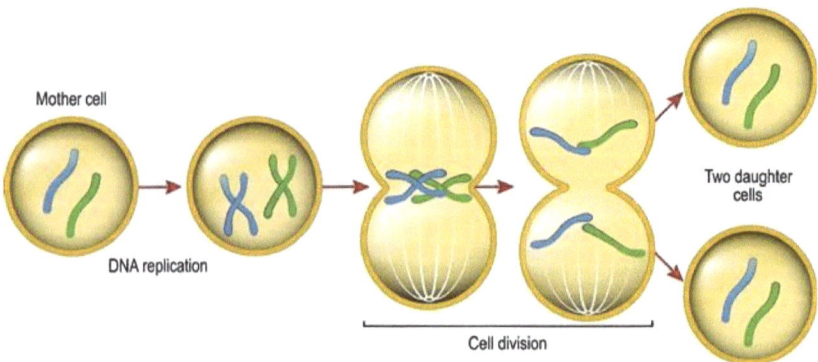

Ref: https://biologywise.com/difference-between-mitosis-meiosis

Although the 23 pairs are the normal complement for humans, very occasionally things go wrong and some people unfortunately are born having an extra (or an absence) of a chromosome. For example, someone who has Down's syndrome has an extra chromosome No. 21. This is known as a Trisomy disorder.

Syndrome	Abnormality
Down's	Extra No.21
Turner's	Absence of Y in No.23
Paton's	Extra No.13
Klinefelter's	Extra X in No.23

Ref https://www.betterhealth.vic.gov.au/health/conditionsandtreatments/trisomy-disorders

Because of the increased study in the genetic nature of diseases, specific areas of chromosomes can now be designated as disease relevant ones as shown below for Chromosomes 1 and 2 respectively.

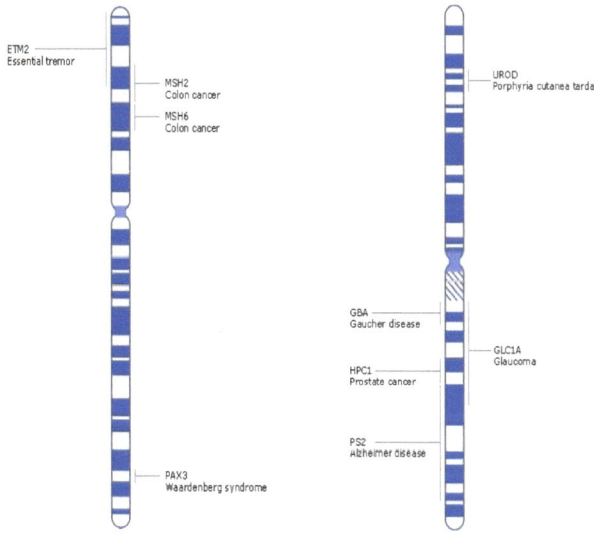

Ref: https://www.ncbi.nlm.nih.gov/books/NBK22266/

https://www.genome.gov/about-genomics/fact-sheets/Chromosome-Abnormalities-Fact-Sheet

Genetic code errors that result in diseases

Because genes are codes that lead to the formation of proteins, it follows that an error in the DNA code could result in the formation of an incorrect protein that can't function in the required manner. An excellent example of this is the code that produces a protein called haemoglobin that's found in red blood cells. This is a chain of 147 amino acids that is involved in transporting oxygen to cells around the body. The sixth amino acid of haemoglobin is normally glutamic acid (DNA code: GAG) but this is replaced in the mutation by the amino acid valine (DNA code: GTG) which leads to the 147 numbered protein being a different shape to the correct one.

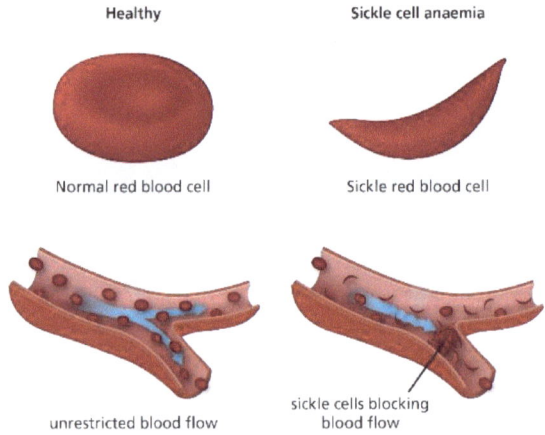

Ref: https://www.yourgenome.org/facts/what-is-sickle-cell-anaemia

This shape difference becomes expressed in the red blood cells themselves giving them a sickle shape rather than the familiar globular shape. The altered blood cells cannot now circulate easily inside the blood capillaries, and the body's vital organs will therefore be deprived of the oxygen they need to function properly.

There are several other single gene mutation derived diseases that humans can succumb to depending upon whether the gene is what's known as **dominant** or **recessive**. The former is expressed from only one mutant version derived from a parent, while the latter requires two versions of the same mutant derived from each parent.

https://learn.genetics.utah.edu/content/disorders/singlegeneeg/

Cancer protection

The obvious main hazard of genetic mutation is that it can result in uncontrolled cellular growth, leading to the formation of tumours that can spread and generate secondary growths in other parts of the body. These are the cancers that many people rightfully dread, because their onset usually marks the beginning of a long term battle against the disease. What is not generally appreciated, however, is that humans have a natural suppressor gene called the TP53 Gene, which is constantly on the guard for such genetic defects, and which usually leads to the rapid death of the harmful cell (called Apoptosis). It is considered that over half of human cancers only arise once the TP53 gene itself has been mutated to inactivate it.

https://www.whatisbiotechnology.org/index.php/science/summary/p53-gene/

Interestingly, elephants are known to have twenty copies of the TP53 gene which is one reason why it's very rare for them to succumb to the disease, whereas humans have just the one copy.

https://the-gist.org/2015/12/why-elephants-never-seem-to-get-cancer/

Genetic factors that control body development

Some genes lead to the production of proteins that are themselves regulators of other genes. An excellent example are a group called the Homeobox (or Hox) genes, which direct how body parts are constructed in the correct head-to-tail order. These are ancient genes that control the body plan of **all creatures** from the embryo level and have been doing so since eukaryotic life first arose around 1.5 billion years ago. For this reason they are defined as being 'highly conserved genes' meaning that they haven't changed much over the eons, although they may reside on different chromosomes depending upon species variety. The diagram below shows how closely similar the plan is followed for both a human and a fly.

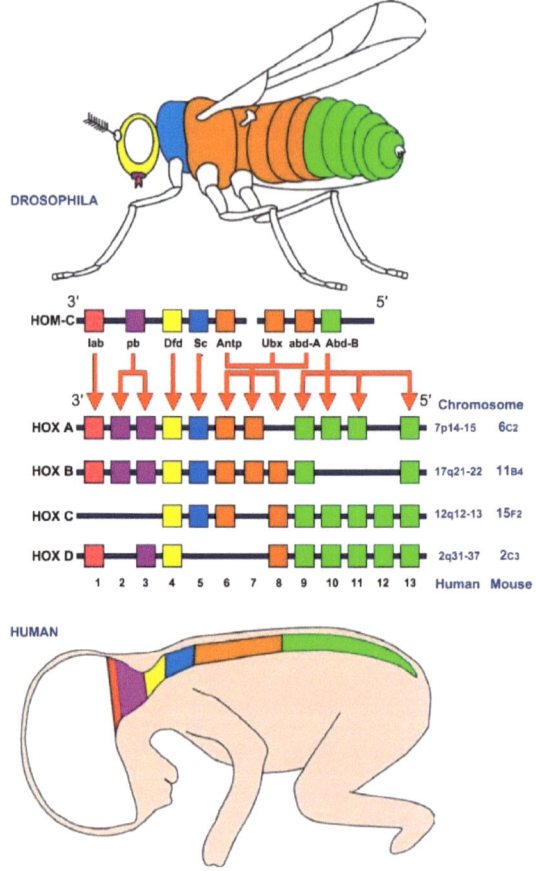

Ref: https://socratic.org/biology/reproduction-development/hox-genes

Homeobox genes video: https://www.youtube.com/watch?v=xHFF8R1XU6g

Genetic Toolkit video: https://www.youtube.com/watch?v=mxJ1E7-Yie0

This is the main reason why the early embryos of widely differing creatures are very similar in their form and appearance:

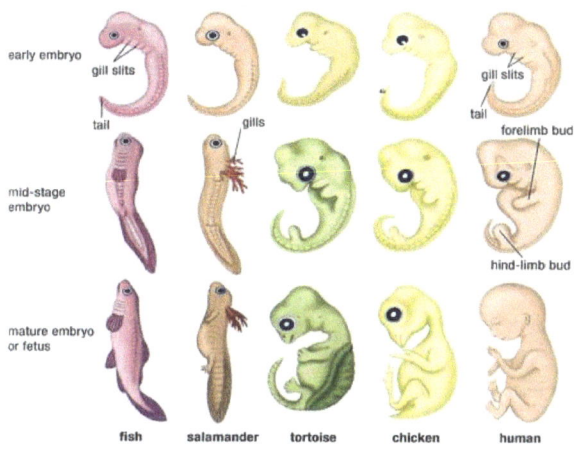

Ref: https://microbenotes.com/evolutionary-embryology/

The evolutionary significance of sex

Humans are just one example of a eukaryotic species that depends upon sexual union between a male and female to produce their offspring. In fact 99% of all eukaryotes use this form of coupling to propagate their species. Evidence for the physical act of copulation has been traced back to a species of armoured fish living 385 million years ago:

https://www.nationalgeographic.com/news/2014/10/141019-fossil-fish-evolution-sex-fertilization/

https://www.sapiens.org/column/origins/sexual-evolution-pleasure/

In contrast, simple lifeforms such a bacteria, amoeba and some plants use an **asexual** method to regenerate exact copies of themselves using the aforementioned process of cellular division called **Mitosis**. This means that the genome of the progeny remains largely the same and no significant variation in their characterisation is possible over several generations.

When it comes to humans, however, it is obvious from experience that two parents will produce children having widely differing features from their parents and who are also dissimilar to one another. The main reason is that a mixing of chromosome segments occurs between parental genes (called a

Crossing Over of genes) to eventually provide a unique egg for the female which is then fertilised by an equally unique sperm from the male to result in a unique child. In effect, half the (mixed) chromosomes from the mother will have been coupled with half the (mixed) chromosomes of the father.

The process that leads to this mixing is called **Meiosis with crossover**, and leads to the production of two parental **gametes** (i.e. a sperm and an egg) which combine to form on conception a **zygote** which then undergoes standard mitotic growth to eventually become a baby. The male gamete is produced in the testes, while the female egg is produced in the ovaries. Because gametes contains single chromosomes which are ready to be paired off they are defined as being **haploid** cells, while a normal paired cell is defined as being **diploid**. Generally any cells in the body that are not directly involved in gamete production are known as **somatic** cells.

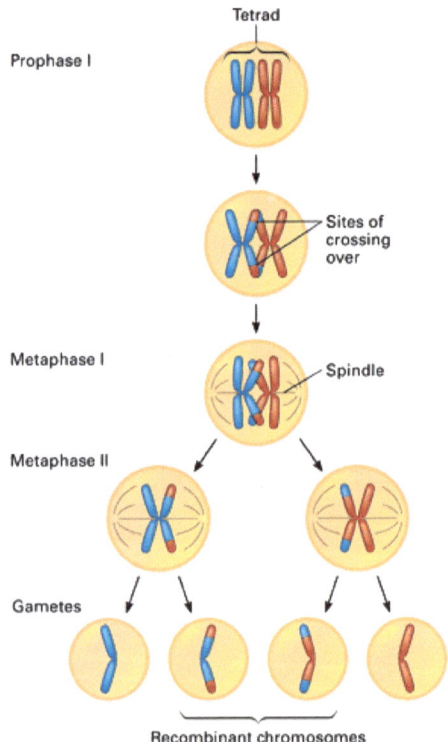

Ref: https://bodell.mtchs.org/OnlineBio/BIOCD/text/chapter9/concept9.6.html

So the question that arises is **why** has this elaborate gene shuffling procedure evolved for eukaryotic life to regenerate itself? The answer is that it allows for variability to occur within each generation to make it easier to withstand any environmental pressures that will impact upon it - i.e. the very pressures that have led to the huge diversity of complex life that we see today. For example, the evolution of the great range of dog species from their ancestral wolf described earlier could never have happened if sexual mixing of genetic information hadn't taken place. A further benefit from sexual reproduction comes from the reduction of harmful genetic mutations that might otherwise result from the asexual generation of daughter cells.

http://www.bbc.co.uk/earth/story/20160704-the-real-reasons-why-we-have-sex

https://phys.org/news/2015-01-affirms-sexual-reproduction-mutations.html

Plants are also eukaryotic in origin, and may therefore also rely on sexual union for reproduction purposes. This is most apparent for bisexual flowering plants, in which pollen that are found in the plant's stamen are equivalent to male gametes, while female ovules are found in the plant's carpal. The union between the two can occur in a variety of ways.

Video: https://www.youtube.com/watch?v=R8_ScKzLAfE

5. Epilogue

The foregoing sections will have revealed how complex life eventually emerged on Earth over billions of years from an environment driven agenda in combination with a number of unpredictable events that has led to the huge range of life that we currently share with on our planet. As far as is known, no other life exists in our solar system, and none has so far been detected elsewhere in the universe. This is a direct consequence of the fact that we live in just the right proximity to our sun called the Goldilocks Zone where it is 'not too hot, and not too cold' for water and life to exist. This location is also known as the habitable zone, and astronomers are currently on the look-out for other planets (called Exoplanets) outside of the solar system which are situated in similar habitable zones.

Video: discovered planet: https://www.youtube.com/watch?v=jbZD4wYztC4

How might the knowledge of the emergence of life on Earth be extrapolated to life existing elsewhere in the universe? Some important factors will remain constant. For example, any possible alien life is also very likely to be carbon based, because this element is the only one that can form strong bonds with itself, leading to chained linkages, which is why such long compounds such as DNA and RNA can exist in the first place. And these were present in the very first lifeforms on Earth, bacteria and archaea, and a discussion of how these are likely to have resulted from pre-life self-replicating molecules was presented early on in this book. But there is another possibility - a theory called Panspermia, which posits that life might have been 'seeded' on this planet from elsewhere, the implication being that bacterial and archaeal life may themselves have had an extra-terrestrial origin. Alternatively, extra-terrestrial RNA-type molecules may have been the seeding factor.

https://www.panspermia.org/intro.htm

However, the flaw with the idea of Panspermia is that it merely transfers the life's origin conundrum to another location! But if future probes, for example those going to Mars, do succeed in discovering bacterial life similar to those on Earth this would certainly enhance the possibility of Panspermia being a realistic proposition.

But of course we're far more interested in knowing if **intelligent life** exists elsewhere in the universe. From the evidence presented in this book the evolution of complex lifeforms such as animals only came about from a chance encounter of an archaea species with a bacterial one which ended up with the former engulfing the latter (i.e. endosymbiosis). Gene transfer from the latter to the former eventually transformed the bacterial entity into mitochondria that was an essential step into utilising the energy derived from food and oxygen and lead to the much larger creatures that exist today, ourselves included. This encounter happened only once during Earth's five billion year history, so how likely would it be for a similar process to occur on another planet? In my opinion it's very unlikely, but the saving grace is that there are literally billions of planets in the universe, so that even with such a low probability, the chances of intelligent life existing out there are still high. What form could this life take? We've seen how in order to enable logical thought a creature would need to have high processing power - which in biological terms would be mean having a large brain.

What would such a creature use this power for? From our own experience it would probably be used for learning about their environment and creating tools to make their lives better. And if they then wished to explore their own star system they could use their intelligence to build probes much like we humans do today. But in order to do that, they would additionally require manual dexterity to enable the putting together of intricate electronic equipment - in other words employing something like the appendages that we have - i.e. hands with fingers and thumbs! The creature would also need to be mobile, so a minimum of two legs with feet would be required. The inescapable conclusion one can draw is that any space travelling intelligent life that we may encounter in the future is likely to have evolved into the humanoid form in order to bring all these attributes together. It would be of great interest to see if this scenario turns out to be correct in any future encounter with them.

Summary

As should be very apparent by now, all life on Earth is related to one another through DNA, and this is made obvious by the fact that humans share their DNA with cats to the tune of 90%, mice and cows (80%), zebrafish (71%) and chickens (60%). If life hadn't emerged from a single ancient ancestor known as LUCA (i.e. Last Universal Common Ancestor) such facts could not be easily explained.

https://phys.org/news/2018-12-luca-universal-common-ancestor.html

The significant difference that great apes have 48 diploid chromosomes while humans have only 46 (i.e. 23 from each parent) by virtue of the combination of two ape chromosomes to form the No.2 chromosome in humans should also be noted. The ubiquitous nature of chromosomes in all eukaryotic life can be appreciated from the table below:

Organism	Chromosome number
Agrodiaetus butterfly	268
Red viscacha rat	102
Woodland hedgehog	88
Pitcher plant	78
Dog (and Grey wolf)	78
Red deer	68
Elephant	56
Strawberry	56
Cotton	52
Gorilla	**48**
Potato	48
Tobacco	48
Human	**46**
Dolphin	44
Peanut	40
Pig	38
Tiger	38
Earthworm	36
Pistachio	30
Giraffe	30
Tomato	24
Snail	24
Citrus fruits	18
Kangaroo	16
Cucumber	14
Fruit fly	8
Indian muntjac	6/7*
Mosquito	6
Jack jumper ant	2/1

*The muntjac is a small deer; 6 is for the female, and 7 for the male

Ref: https://en.wikipedia.org/wiki/List_of_organisms_by_chromosome_count

The remarkable small number of chromosomes occurring in the Indian muntjac has been determined to have been caused by multiple fusions of chromosomes similar to the 2 for 1 that occurred from apes to humans:

https://io9.gizmodo.com/this-prehistoric-pocket-deer-has-fewer-chromosomes-than-1705706404

And to conclude, below is a reminder of how much DNA we share with other similar eukaryote cousins:

DNA similarity to humans

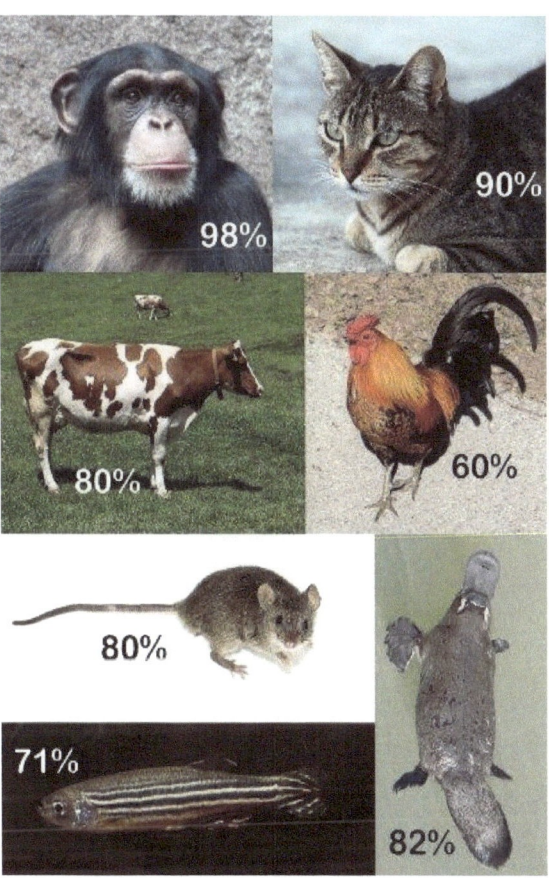

Ref: https://genetics.thetech.org/ask-a-geneticist/human-seal-shared-dna

www.ingramcontent.com/pod-product-compliance
Lightning Source LLC
Chambersburg PA
CBHW040239220526
45473CB00001B/298